RENAL DIET

A Complete Beginner's Guide to Live Healthy With Healthy
Kidneys

(Ultimate Guide to Equip Its Reader With Knowledge)

Pedro Elkins

Published by Alex Howard

Renal Diet: A Complete Beginner's Guide to Live Healthy With Healthy Kidneys (Ultimate Guide to Equip Its Reader With Knowledge)

ISBN 978-1-989891-90-2

Legal & Disclaimer

The information contained in this book is not designed to replace or take the place of any form of medicine or professional medical advice. The information in this book has been provided for educational and entertainment purposes only.

Table of contents

Part 1

Introduction

It is strongly recommended that people with renal impairment strictly follow a renal or renal diet to drastically reduce the amount of toxic compounds or wastes in the bloodstream. Toxic compounds, or rather, wastes in the blood, as many people call it, usually come from the type of food and liquids consumed. If a kidney is compromised or not functioning optimally, it simply means that the kidneys will not filter or dispose of waste as they should. If a toxic substance is not removed or left in the bloodstream, it is very harmful because it can negatively affect the patient's electrolyte level. Strict adherence to a renal diet greatly improves renal function and also reduces the tendency of the kidney to develop complete renal failure.

What exactly is a renal diet? This is a diet that contains little sodium, phosphorus and, of course, protein. A kidney diet also teaches you how important it is to consume only high quality protein and limit fluid intake. In some cases, patients are asked to also reduce the intake of potassium and calcium. As humans, we all have different body systems. Therefore, it is very important that a patient has a personal diabetic kidney. The renal dietitian will develop the ideal diet that is perfect for the patient, or rather develop a diet that meets the nutritional needs of the patient. When a patient begins to notice a worsening renal function, it is now difficult to eliminate protein and mineral wastes from the body. If the kidneys are compromised, it would be even more difficult for the kidneys to eliminate toxins from the bloodstream. As I mentioned earlier, each renal diet recipe in a patient must be different due to the differences in our body, but all the nutrients that a patient with kidney damage needs to reduce are proteins, phosphorus, potassium and, of course, sodium-rich foods . In this book, you will learn how to start preparing a healthy meal for the kidneys and, of course, to maintain a healthy lifestyle. The type of food you eat and drink when you have renal dysfunction has the full potential of having a great impact on your well-being. If this lifestyle is constantly followed, your treatment will definitely be more effective.

Let us not forget the fact that a good meal not only provides good health to patients with renal insufficiency but to all people. But it is inevitable and very important for patients with chronic kidney disease. Even if a patient undergoes renal dialysis treatment, it is not absolute to remove bodily wastes from the bloodstream. It is advisable to maintain close contact with your personal kidney dietitian to find the ideal nutritional plan that best suits your body system and also help you select some of your favorite foods that are good for you. In most cases, your personal diet plan will depend on your age, weight, preferred foods, type of dialysis treatments and other conditions such as diabetes, heart failure and, of course, your blood pressure. This cookbook was designed to meet your nutritional needs, but may not meet the nutritional needs of other specific patients. In general, it is accepted that people with kidney disease should be careful with the type of food and the intake of certain nutrients. It is expected that you only eat foods that are easily digestible. If you strictly adhere to the nutritional plan prescribed by your personal kidney dietitian, you will get a much better result. Keep in mind that calories are crucial to enrich your body with the energy you need for your daily activities. It is the duty of your renal diabetologist to help you plan your meal. The food should contain the right amount and the right amount of calories from different food sources to help your body stay strong and healthy.

- The most important food classes
- Protein helps develop new body tissues and repair damaged ones. There are several foods that you consume and that contain protein. Now milk, eggs, lean meat, poultry and, of course, seafood are the ideal and healthy source of protein. Now we have bread, cereals and vegetables for carbohydrates. One thing about vegetables is that they are mainly carbohydrates, but they also contain traces of protein nutrients.
- Carbohydrates strengthen the body with energy; It comes in the form of starch and sugar / glucose. The various main sources of carbohydrates are corn, fruits, bread, vegetables and cereals. If a patient

suffers from diabetes, care should be taken with carbohydrate intake to control blood sugar.

- Fat is another form of energy source, but in concentrated form, fat essentially adds moisture, flavor and a certain amount of calories to our diet. It is mostly included in a nutritional plan for a patient with chronic kidney disease, providing the body with the essential calories that help it increase or even maintain body weight. If the patient is overweight and wants to lose weight, his nutritionist or doctor can take him on a low-fat diet. If you are the type that is cautious in terms of fat content, there are certain types of fat that are recommended for you.

- Potassium: this mineral regulates nerve and muscle function. Potassium is generally available as it is found in almost all foods. Now here are some foods that are very rich in potassium and are bananas, avocados, beans, cereals and peas, milk and nuts, oranges, winter squash, potatoes, tomatoes and dried fruits. The frequency with which these foods rich in potassium can be consumed, or what portions the body can tolerate at any given time, depends on the needs of your person.

- Calcium and Phosphorus: these are essential minerals that work hand in hand in the body's system. They help keep bones healthy and strong. Now there would be a problem if the kidneys have difficulty filtering phosphorus. Then the phosphorus levels in the blood would become high. If you have high levels of calcium and phosphorus in the blood, it will cause bone disease and calcification of the arteries and organs of the blood, including the heart. Do not worry, there is a way out, the patient will be given a constant intake of medications that bind to phosphorus and will be on a diet, consuming foods with low phosphorus content. You can find phosphorus in almost all foods that contain a certain amount of phosphorus, but you can find them more frequently in dairy products such as cheese, milk and yogurt, nuts, chocolate, dried beans and even coke drinks. Your doctor and a good renal dietitian can help you reconcile your dietary intake with your medication.

- Sodium: this mineral helps regulate body fluids. The consumption of sodium-rich foods can interfere with the regulation of body fluids in severe kidney disease. Most sodium-rich foods are processed foods. These include smoked fish or meat, bacon, processed cheese, ham, sausages and cheese. Snacks like cucumbers, pretzels, salted nuts, corn and chips also contain a lot of sodium. It is not necessary that all foods high in sodium have a salty taste. Some foods high in sodium have no salty taste. Examples of these foods include tomato sauce, canned soups, mustard, condiments, meat tenderizers, some spices, meat sauces, processed or packaged foods, and fast foods. It is better to prepare your own food because if you prepare your own food from the beginning, you have all the opportunities to control the amount of sodium you use.

- Healthy consumption of spices
- It is very important to use only pure spices, not spices made with salt. Some of the recommended spices are fresh lemon or lime juice, fresh garlic, garlic powder, paprika, pepper, onion powder, just the right amount of green pepper, onion, vinegar and wine. You should refrain from spices that consist of potassium chloride. Not all salt substitutes are made up of sodium. Many of them contain a good amount of potassium. To be honest, potassium turns out to be more dangerous to your health like a salt. Here are some ideal suggestions for mixing your spices with specific foods:

- Sauces Bay Leaf beef
- Spice beef
- Eggs fish
- Fruits
- Vegetables
- Beverages
- Baked products
- Desserts Basil lamb
- Fish
- Veal
- Cinnamon chicken
- Pork
- Baked products
- Beverages
- Vegetables

- Cloves beef
- Pork fruits Curry (non-salted) beef
- Chicken
- Lamb
- Eggs Dill chicken
- Vegetables Ginger chicken
- Meats
- Poultry
- Mustard Powder meats
- Vegetables Parsley beef
- Salads
- Sauces Rosemary beef
- Turkey Sage meats
- Stuffing
- Vegetables Savory egg dishes meats
- Rice
- Vegetables Tarragon chicken
- Vegetables Thyme fish

For the perfect crush or rub leaf-type herbs so as to release their total flavor, use vegetable. Don't forget herbs that spices should not overwhelm the taste of your food, so it is best you add them in small quantity. Nonetheless, we all know that salt brings the best out of flavors or increases flavors; you may use your initiative to slightly add more of a spice than a standard written in this recipe.

Please Note

Sometimes meal planning is not always rosy, it can be challenging but your will to stay healthy might overcome the challenge. In this cookbook you will learn how to mix recipes in your meal planning for chronic kidney disease patients.

Please note that the meal plan given to you in the cookbook have been estimated and calculated to provide nourishment, your body can tolerate the quantity of the stated food compound bellow per day:

- 2000 calories

- 70grams protein

- 2 grams sodium

- 2 grams potassium

- 1000 mg phosphorus

- You can be sure that the recipes you will find in this book improve your culinary skills and help you prepare delicious and healthy foods that are good for your body system. You can contact your renal nutritionist at any time to help you choose the ideal ingredients, as you need to know how much these ingredients can support your body. The complete recipe has been researched and analyzed to make sure it contains the following nutrients:

- Calories
- Carbohydrates
- Protein
- Fat
- Sodium
- Potassium and phosphorus

And you can be sure that the recipe you will find in this book has also been researched and analyzed for the exchange of kidney and kidney diabetics. We use the National Lists of Exchange of Renal Diets. (For more information on these lists, contact your personal nutritionist.)

The national renal diet exchange lists include a "salt exchange" that contains up to 250 milligrams of sodium. In this cookbook you will find recipes that use this salt exchange. We have carefully researched and analyzed these recipes for kidney and kidney diabetic replacement. Keep in mind that you may need to consult your nutritionist since some of these recipes may have a high sugar content, which is not good for diabetics. We have carefully labeled these recipes with the note "Not suitable for patients with diabetes". Please keep this in mind. We have calculated these recipes below:

• Practor Care

• Neutri Practor 6000

• SanDiego, California, 1990; Food Processor II, ESHA Research, Salem, Oregon; and Pennington's"Bowes & Church's Food Values of Portions Commonly Used," The 16th edition.

What Is Organic Food And The Benefits Of Organic Food

What is Organic Food? Organic food is something that has come about from people like you and I seeing and learning about the effects of highly processed foods being provided to us by big corporations. The definition of "Organic" when it comes to Food is regulated and defined by the USDA, specifically the National Organic Program also referred to as NOP. This article will discuss the different definitions of "Organic" in different industries along with supplying you with concrete information to find a Ωuality organic grower.

NOP defines "Organic" as follows: "Organic is a labeling term that indicates that the food or other agricultural product has been produced through approved methods that integrate cultural, biological, and mechanical practices that foster cycling of resources, promote ecological balance, and conserve biodiversity. Synthetic fertilizers, sewage sludge, irradiation, and genetic engineering may not be used."

The NOP lets certified growers use a label which reads "USDA ORGANIC". You may also see "100% Organic" listed around the USDA ORGANIC label. 100% Organic means that every ingredient in said product is certified organic. USDA Organic means at least 95% of the ingredients are certified organic. You may also see "Made with Organic Ingredients" means at least 70% of the ingredients are certified organic, BUT they can't use the USDA ORGANIC label on said product.

The USDA National Organic Program has control over how food growers and manufactures can become certified and they supply the standards on what inputs can and can't be used in a product. The NOP does not manage or regulate the manufacturers of inputs, for instance fertilizers or specific compounds, only what they will allow in said inputs in any certified organic product or used in a certified growing operation.

Back in 1997 a non-profit company was formed called Organic Materials Institute (OMRI), that provides organic certifiers, growers, manufacturers, and suppliers an independent review of products intended for use in certified organic production, handling, and processing. The majority of Organic Food manufactures and producers rely on OMRI for available inputs that meet or exceed the NOP Standards.

You go to the nursery or big box store to get some garden or lawn fertilizer and you see listed on a bag "Organic Fertilizer". You may say, "looks great" because Gardening 101 says I only want to use an organic fertilizer on my organic garden. Sounds great, right? Here is where the problem of trying to do the right thing can turn bad. The first thing to realize if that "Organic" listed on a food item is completely different then "Organic" listed on anything else such as fertilizer, compost, soils, mulch, or any other product you will find at a nursery.

There are more than a dozen ways to define "Organic" and they are all right depending on the perspective. A chemist or chemical manufacture may define "Organic" as any compound that contains a Carbon (C) and

Hydrogen (H) bond. An organic compound can consist of a large class of gaseous, li?uid, or solid chemical compounds whose molecules contain carbon. The point is that anything outside "Food" has a completely different meaning for organic.

Don't be fooled by some local or national grower that says "I'm not certified organic, but we don't use any pesticides or harmful chemicals on our produce". There is no way to prove what they are saying without someone checking their farm out for problems, but when you hear this ASK QUESTIONS! Specifically, ask them exactly what they use by brand and name as inputs in their growing operations. Many of these farmers have been doing it a particular way for years and have a mindset that if it was OK to do forty years ago it must be a good thing to do today.

When you talk to any grower ask them specifically what fertilizer they use, specifically by brand and name. If you want to know if it is approved for organic gardens check to see if this fertilizer is listed on the OMRI website. There are many so-called experts out there that want to sell you something, but finding someone who can help you put it all together for your specific garden is challenging. When you are asking for help make sure you specifically ask if they are speaking "fact" or "opinion". If they say fact ask them where you could find the source of these facts.

How To Prepare For Usmc Boot Camp By Eating The Right Type Of Food

When you search on how to prepare for USMC boot camp, you'll mostly read about stuff for physical fitness and the first thing that comes to mind is exercise or workout routine. Keep in mind that physical fitness involves your diet. A healthy, balanced diet always goes hand-in-hand with exercise. Eat a proper diet before you enter the Marines so that you will be prepared for the demanding basic training you would have to go through.

One way on how to prepare for USMC boot camp when it comes to diet and nutrition is by learning about protein and carbohydrates. Protein is one of the three major classes of food or source of food energy that is abundant in animal-derived foods like meat and some vegetables like legumes. Forget about protein shakes, what you need is real protein. Don't believe everything you see on ads. What does protein do? It helps build muscle and it strengthens your body. When you strengthen your muscles, you lessen the chance of you getting injured during training. Increase the amount of protein you eat so that you'll be boot camp ready. Stick to lean meat and trim the fat.

What about carbohydrates? You need carbs as your source of energy but make sure you are eating the healthier alternatives. Avoid donuts, cereals and other sugary stuff. Stick to whole-grained pasta, bread and rice. There are plenty of available choices in your local grocery store. Don't forget your fruits and vegetables!

High Cholesterol Foods - Are They The Major Reasons For High Cholesterol?

High cholesterol foods should be avoided mostly and should be restricted in your diet, whether you already have been diagnosed with high cholesterol or not. You may be affected and not know, because there may not be any major obvious symptoms.

Here is a list of the most common high cholesterol foods:

Fast food and junk food

Fast food and junk food are usually high in cholesterol, salt, calories and sugar. Some very bad fats called trans fats are usually found in fast food. Trans fats are by-products of hydrogenated oil. They behave like saturated fats when they get in the body. They clog up the human arteries and cause plaque to build up contributing to heart disease and stroke symptoms.

Some people believe that if they exercise more they can eat fast food or junk food. That's off beam. Exercise will not provide the results you want on its own without diet changes and healthier eating habits.

Fast food does little by way of providing nutrition. They contain all the things that contribute to raising your LDL cholesterol level. Bear in mind that fast food restaurants are not thinking about your nutritional needs when they prepare these foods. Just one meal from a typical fast food restaurant can contain all the total fat and saturated fat quantities experts recommend you have for the day.

How then do you eat your other two meals in the day without consuming too much fat? By the way the excess fat just stores itself in your body and possibly around the arteries. Dangerous.

Now you can understand why fast food and junk food are a major class of high cholesterol foods.

Cheese

Generally, cheese is high in cholesterol. So use genuine low-fat versions if you want to eat cheese. Cheese should be eaten on occasion, not as part of a lifestyle. If you have healthy cookware that enables you to de-fat cheese and other family foods automatically, then you can eat your cake and have it!

Soya versions of cheese are much healthier. Tofu too is.

Milk

Milk is another of foods high in cholesterol. This is because cheese high in the types of fat that produce cholesterol too. Full-fat milk to be precise is, so semi-skimmed and skimmed milk are much better options. Soy milk and rice milk are great replacements.

The Effects Of Fast Food

As the world progresses people do not have time for anything, adults are entirely rapped up in there jobs, as they just want to be successful and give there family a wealthy living and students are now more than ever attending after school classes such as martial arts, singing or dancing lessons. So where does this current living lifestyle leave us with fulfilling our body with the correct nutrients?

Well I can answer this straight away, a huge population of the modern day families are now turning to fast food and ready made meals, as people no longer have time in the day to sit down and cook a meal. But these meals have a devastating effect on not only our body but also our minds. We will now take a look at some major disadvantages from eating this type of food.

The first and most obvious is obesity, it has been stated that one cheeseburger contains more calories than our bodies need to consume in a whole day. Therefore if you make one trip to a fast food outlet and consume 3 burgers, you will be eating a weeks worth of calories in a day. Now imagine you were constantly eating the same meal every day of the week, 3 cheeseburgers a days will equal to 21 cheeseburgers a week, which gives a massive 7 weeks of recommended calories.

Now switch this to a month of eating cheeseburgers and you would have already exceeded half a years of calories and this is not even taking into account the fries or drink.

But besides from putting on weight, obesity can have a major ill effect on your health. It is said that obesity is the major cause of chronic diseases such as diabetes, heart disease and even cancer.

As you probably already know, food directly affects the way in which we think and feel, as junk food is very low in nutritional value and full of preservatives it has led researchers to come to the evaluation that the terrible ingredients can lead to mental disorders such as dyslexia and ADHD.

Eating fast food in moderation is acceptable, eating vegetables and fresh foods should always be your number one priority no matter how busy you may be, your health should be your major concern in life. As no one wishes to spend there time sitting around in a hospital. Remember you only get one life so look after it!

The trouble with fast food

Fast food companies have always gone to great lengths to convince the eating public of the wholesomeness of their food. It's an incredibly profitable business. But, one of the business risks, in a health-conscious age, is having a reputation tainted by thought that your food is unhealthy or, worse, disgusting.

So, typical fast food - in the main - is safe for consumption and may be moderately healthy. But why do we feel unhealthy having eaten it? Compared to a serving of grandma's pot roast where we felt sated and fulfilled, fast food tends to leave us feeling unfulfilled, spiritually.

I have a thesis about food: the only prepared food profitable to us is the food cooked with love. That is, food cooked for a known individual to eat. Food cooked with them in mind. It's food that has soul.

FOOD SHOULD BE PREPARED WITH PRIDE

In the healthiest sense, proud is the cook that makes their food to please the eater. They have a vested interest in everything they do. They want to create it tasty, hygienic, and aesthetic on the plate. They care. They cook their food with love. And they want their food eaten with love and respect for the process.

Fast food, on the other hand, is an unloved child whose parent neither loves the food, their work, nor the receiver of the food. It's made with no soul or spirit. It may fill our bellies and nourish our bodies, but the experience of eating fast food does nothing to nourish our souls.

We ought to become keen observers of how food makes us feel, and although food of itself doesn't make us evil, our practices can sometimes make us feel that way. Feeling bloated or dry in the mouth or queasy are all psychosomatic signs that the experience of eating certain food hasn't been positive. The food hasn't served its nourishing purpose.

THE SERVICE THAT COMES WITH THE FOOD

Whenever we go to takeaway restaurants, not only is the food not cooked with love, it's often not served with love. Patrons are commonly treated as second-class citizens; mainly because the person serving them has no propriety. They've not been trained to care.

Wherever we go in life it pays, as much as possible, to place ourselves in situations and circumstances of good experience. Enriching experience is good for the soul. Placing ourselves in non-enriching experiences, though, leads to a deadening of the soul. The service that comes with the food is just as important as the eating experience is. The service, too, must come with love.

The five classes of wine

Although there are many varieties of each class, the five major classes of wine are as follows:

8Red table wines: More or less red in color, these wines are suited to accompany food. They may be labeled with a generic name (for example, claret) or a varietal name (Cabernet). Or they may represent the grape by its full name - such as Cabernet Sauvignon. Rose wines (pink in color) are also in the red wine class.

White table wines: As the name implies, these are white wines, but the actual color appearing in your glass can range from straw yellow to deep amber. The label usually does not indicate what variety of grape is used so you'll have to hunt a little into the ingredient label on the back of the bottle.

Sparkling wines: As suggested by their name, these wines - red, white or rose- sparkle or bubble. This class includes the champagnes and sparkling burgundies. To get their sparkle, some vintners will use the same type of carbonation used in making soda pop. These are the less expensive varieties. The better sparkling wines, such as champagne, use a natural fermentation process. Some still wines will have a natural state of effervescence, or bubbles, not to be confused with a sparkling wine.

Dessert wine: cream sherry, port, muscatel and sweet vermouth. Dessert wines and aperitif wine can almost share a class, but these four are reserved as strictly dessert wines. Other types of vermouth come under the aperitif class. Dessert wines are sweet tasting, a condition obtained by halting the fermentation process early, so that the juice retains much of its sugar content.

Aperitif wine: the word 'aperitif' meaning appetizer. These wines are usually served chilled before dinner, and are meant to stimulate the appetite. An example of an aperitif wine is Palomino, a pale, dry sherry.

Although they are not designated as a class of wine, the fruit and berry wines usually fall under the dessert wine class.

Campus foods and how protein can help

College is a fun and exciting time in a young person's life. For many of them, it is the first time they are away from their parent's home and making adult decisions on their own. While parents are worried at home about the dangers of drinking, drug, and grades; they worry that their children will not sleep enough or will take on more than they can actually handle. What they may not be concerned with, or what they may forget to talk to their college bound child about, is the campus food.

It is not just a myth that people hit the freshman fifteen, and then some when they enter college. It is a combination of many factors that leaves many of them gaining weight during that first year away from home. One of the major reasons that these students gain weight is due to the campus foods and meal plans offered by most schools.

Campus Foods: Offerings For the Average School

Most schools are making great strides in the campus dining, however, with budget cuts in virtually every school and university across the country, fresh, wholesome and healthy foods are not always easy to come by. In some schools, cafeterias are only open during specific times which may be hard for the student to get to- especially if the student is working in addition to classes. Some schools may offer alternative means for campus food, but not always.

Cafeteria and Other Hot Food Options

Campus foods should not be expected to be gourmet meals - after all, these are cooks working in long, hard shifts in industrial kitchens to churn out a variety of foods for thousands of students and faculty members. These are people who may eat anything put in front of them or may complain and waste the foods that they take. The problem with the cafeteria style, campus foods might be the very way they are cooked and served. Fried foods tend to sit in their grease under heat lamps so they do not congeal. Fresh foods wilt and wither. At the end of the serving period (which may be as long as two hours) the food that is remaining is thrown away and the next meal's foods are prepared and brought back out.

To give this vast amount of food flavor, typically additional sodium is added and that can be an additional problem for weight gain and campus foods.

Grab and Go Food Options

To make accommodations for those students who are not able to get to the cafeterias during their meal serving times, many schools offer a small menu of lesser options that can include sandwiches, fruits and other foods that range from small snacks to more substantial food items. However, most of these foods are high in fat and filled with preservatives.

Campus Foods and Food Plans

Many schools offer a food plan for their students, especially those who are living on campus. These plans usually allow a certain amount of money to be put into the student's account to be used throughout the month. These can be set up as part of the tuition at some schools and will be replenished on certain dates.

For some kids, the concept of budgeting, even their food allotment, can be completely new. They might feast like Henry the Eighth the first week of the month and then live on ketchup, soup,, and ramen noodles for the last week. Those plans don't specify how much can be spent per day or per week nor do they specifically say what the money can be spent on.

Factors Beyond Campus Foods

In addition to the campus foods, weight gain can be caused by other factors. Many of these students are living alone for the first time - they won't always make the best or most adult choices for their foods. Moreover, they are under a lot of stress which can also leave them making poor choices and may lead to increased weight gain.

The American Psychological Association released a study that shows that nearly 75% of adults in the United States feel stressed out and that nearly ½ of those people tend to eat unhealthy foods as a direct result of that stress. One in three is depressed and 42% also feel that the stress has increased since last year (Kimberly Goad Stop Stress for Good. Fitness Magazine. September 2010). That stress tends to lead to an increase in cortisol, the stress hormone that leads to serious weight gain, especially around the belly.

New college students also may start experimenting with alcohol which can also lead to weight gain not only because of the calories that are contained in each drink but because they can lead to a decrease in inhibition.

Making Better Choices in Campus Foods

The best thing a parent can do is to instill healthy eating and living choices in their children before they hit their rebellious teen years and certainly before it is time for them to take off and live on their own. Show them how to choose grilled foods over fried, and that baked, roasted or broiled food choices are also healthier. Show them that they can destroy a perfectly healthy salad by adding cheese or heavy salad dressings. Let them see how to make a healthy food choice out of some limited food selections.

In addition, send your student care packages with easy foods that they can keep - foods that will not go bad and re uire only minimal effort. Send them gift cards for healthy food places so that they are at least getting a meal or two. And, send them Profect, a protein supplement from Protica. Not only is it in a cool, test tube styled package but it is available in a number of refreshing fruit based flavors. It is also high in protein and low in calories and can be consumed in seconds, perfect for the busy student on the go.

Cholesterol medications - understanding the different classes

Diet and exercise are normally the first choice for controlling high cholesterol for many people.

Unfortunately there are some people whose cholesterol does not respond to lifestyle changes but with the help of a cholesterol lowering medication they can easily manage this condition. There are several different classes of cholesterol drugs and in most cases your doctor can help prescribe the one that will work best for you.

LDL cholesterol, also known as low density lipoprotein, is the reason many of these drugs exist. LDL cholesterol is the primary culprit in the formation of arterial pla ue. Pla ue deposits can cause blockages and clots which are a major factor for heart disease and strokes. There are four classes of cholesterol drugs whose main function is to lower LDL levels in the blood stream. These include Statins, Bile Acid Binding Resins, Absorption Inhibitors, and Fibrates. While they work very well they also can have some discomforting side affects for some people, usually of the stomach and digestive system variety. Some people experience cramps, constipation, nausea, and bloating.

Another area of concern with high cholesterol is triglycerides. Triglycerides are fats that come from both animal and plant food sources. In particular saturated fat has been shown in scientific studies to raise blood LDL cholesterol levels more then dietary food cholesterol. Statins, Absorption Inhibitors, and Fibrates moderate and reduce the amount of triglycerides that find their way into the circulatory system.

Another side to the cholesterol equation is HDL, or high density lipoprotein, cholesterol. This is known as the good cholesterol and its primary purpose is to remove excess LDL cholesterol from the blood stream and deliver it to the liver where it is excreted from the body. While Statins, Absorption Inhibitors, and Fibrates are the primary drugs that do this the increase is not large. But in the battle against coronary artery disease every little gain is considered a victory.

There are a number of different drug companies making these types of drugs which can be found under many recognizable names, including Lipitor. The current advertising campaigns in all media types have ingrained many of these drug names in our collective conscious. Your doctor is the best source of information when it comes to deciding which drug will work best for you. It is also important to let your doctor know if you experience any side affects. With the multitude of drugs to choose from your doctor should be able to find one that works well without the side affects.

What are the major problems of being overweight?

Obesity is becoming a major epidemic across the developed world, in Britain alone it is estimated that more than half the adult population is overweight.

So when would a doctor class a patient as being obese? This is defined as someone who weighs 30% more than the acceptable upper limit taking their height, age and sex into account.

The harsh reality is that there is no instant cure for this "disease" the only way to reduce your weight to a more healthy level is through diet and exercise. By reducing the amount of energy we consume in the form of food and in particular fatty food it is possible to achieve this goal.

The effects of obesity on health can be devastating just some of these potential problems are listed below:

1. Painful, aching legs

2. Swelling of the ankles

3. Shortness of breath

4. Damage to the joints which can cause osteoarthritis particularly in the knees and hips.

For those who are very overweight the problems become even more serious:

1. High blood pressure

2. Diabetes

3. Gout

4. Angina

5. Arthritis

All of these illnesses will only become more serious as time passes unless there is an effort made to reduce weight.

Many people will say that they are overweight because it runs in their family or they have some kind of hormone problem or they have a very slow metabolic rate. These statements are very rarely the true cause of obesity. It is true, obesity can often be seen in whole families but it has more to do with older generations passing on unhealthy eating habits to the younger family members.

There is no need for anyone to take drastic measures in an attempt to lose weight. The answer is relatively simple reduce the amount of fat in your diet and eat more foods which are carbohydrates. Two people who consume the same amount of calories, one with a diet high in carbohydrates such as pasta, rice, oats etc. and the other with a diet high in fat i.e. pies, cakes, crisps, pasties, sausages etc. Which is more likely to be obese? The answer is obvious.

Some diets exclude carbohydrates completely this is not the correct way to lose weight effectively. Recommendations state that approximately 50% of our energy should come from carbohydrates and only around 35% from fats.

The only way to lose weight in a way which will ensure that it does not return is with a low fat diet and regular exercise. By doing this the weight loss will be slower but more effective in the long term.

The Medical Significance Of The Arachnida Class Of The Arthropods

The class Arachnida is a group of more than 100,000 species, including spiders, scorpions, ticks and mites. Most arachnids are adapted to kill prey with poison galnds, stingers, or fangs. Like crustaceans, arachnids have a body that is divided into a cephalothorax and an abdomen.

Attached to the Cephalothorax are 4 pairs of legs, a pair of Chelicerae, and a pair of appendages called pedipalps. The pedipalps aid in chewing; in some species pedipalps are specialized to perform other functions. Arachnids undergo incomplete metamorphosis. Class Arachnida includes 3 orders of medical importance:

1. Order Scorpions

2. Order Araneae (spiders)

3. Order Acari (ticks and mites)

Scorpions

The scorpions are familiar group of arachnids whose pedipalps are modified into pincers. Scorpions use these pincers to handle their food and tear it apart. The venomous stings of scorpions are used mainly to stun their prey and less commonly in self-defense. The sting is located in the terminal segment of the body, which is slender toward the end. The elongated, jointed abdomens of scorpions are distinctive; in most chelicerates, the abdominal segments are more or less fused together and appear as a single unit. The adults of this order of arachnids range in size from 1 to 18 centimeters. There are some 1200 species of scorpions, all terrestrial, which occur throughout the world, although they are common in tropical, subtropical, and desert regions. The courtship of scorpions is elaborate, with the spermatophores being fixed to a substrate by the male and then picked up subse❓uently by the female. The young are born alive, with 1 to 95 in a given liter. Scorpions differ from spiders in two ways.

Scorpions have greatly enlarged pedipalps, which they hold in a forward position. They also have a large stinger on the last segment of the abdomen. Most scorpions hide during the day and hunt at night. Scorpions seize their prey with their pincerlike pedipalps. Then the fang injects paralyzing venom, the chelicerae tear the prey,, the animal is ingested, and digestion begins. Only a few species have a sting that may be fetal to humans. They do not sting a man unless attacked.

Pathogenicity

The local symptoms of bite include severe pain, inflammation and swelling. Sweating, nausea and vomiting are common systemic symptoms. Muscular spasm and convulsions can occur in severe cases. Fatal outcome is caused by respiratory failure, pulmonary edema and shock.

Control

Spraying of insecticides

Spiders

There are about 25,000 named species of spiders (order Araneae). These animals play a major role in all terrestrial ecosystems, where they are particularly important as predators of insects and other small animals. Spiders hunt their prey or catch it in webs. The silk of the webs is formed from a fluid protein that is forced out of spinnerets, modified appendages on the posterior portion of the spider's abdomen. Spiders have poison glands leading through their chelicerae, which are pointed and used to bite and paralyze prey. Some members of this order, such as the black widow spider (Latrodectus mactans), Australia black widow spider (Latrodectus seville), caracurt (latrodectus tredicimguttatus), brown recluse (Loxosceles reclusa), tarantula (Lycosa singoriensis), have bites that are poisonous to humans and other large mammals.

Discovering real food

All natural, totally organic, made with real ingredients, nothing artificial, nonfat, whole grain, source of omega 3's. Of course we wouldn't put anything in our mouths if it were not real food, right? What else are we eating if not real foods? The answer: food-like substitutes, imitations, products stuck in a box with a fancy label making health claims. Real food is out there and it is important that we are able to recognize it when we see it. Eating the right foods is imperative to maintaining health and vitality. So lets get back to the basics of why we eat food. What is a real food?

First and foremost, real food sustains life and maintains health. It is non-toxic, it can be eaten without processing, it is digested easily, and it is naturally appealing to our senses. Real food is provided by nature in a form that supplies every nutritional re🞑uirement for the body. These re🞑uirements include glucose, protein, fatty acids, vitamins (enzymes), minerals, and water. Let's talk for a moment about why we need these and where we get them.

Carbohydrates - These are a class of foods that include starches and sugars and come from the plant kingdom. Our energy is ultimately derived from the sugar glucose, which is a simple carbohydrate. The problem with carbohydrates in the American diet is that on average the majority of our food is highly processed, refined carbohydrates, mostly made from wheat and corn, with little to no nutrient value. People tend to overeat these causing weight gain and health problems. Michael Pollen, author of In Defense of Food, says "Sugar as it is ordinarily found in nature -in fruits and some vegetables -gives us a slow-release form of energy accompanied by minerals and all sorts of crucial micronutrients we can get nowhere else." The bulk of our diet should be in the form of carbohydrates, namely those from fresh, raw plant sources.

Proteins - The body uses proteins for growth, replacement and repair of tissue. Dr. Joel Robbins, of Living Health Concepts, says that "since protein is not utilized as fuel and since after the age of weaning our biggest demand for protein in structure building is over, our need for protein is very little." The body cannot use protein in its original state, so it breaks it down into amino acids, which are the building blocks of protein. Most people think of meat when they think of proteins. But did you know that the 8 essential amino acids needed by the body for the production of proteins are found in a variety of fruits, vegetables, sprouts, whole grains, nuts and seeds? Because the blood and liver provide an amino acid pool from which the body can draw, it is not necessary to have a complete protein at every meal. But some of us have been "killing the fatted calf" for breakfast, lunch, and dinner every day.

Fats - For years the food industry has marketed low fat, nonfat, reduced fat foods claiming that fats are bad for us. Fats are absolutely necessary in our diets, and studies are now showing that a lack of healthy fats, especially omega 3 fatty acids, is actually detrimental to our health. Fats are used for aiding in the assimilation of fat-soluble vitamins. They are also used for padding and insulation, making hormones and aiding metabolic processes, and they are a source of heat and energy when carbohydrates are not readily available. Fats occur naturally in plants. However, the American diet has been flooded with harmful fats including hydrogenated fats, heated fats, saturated fats, and free oils. In his book The Raw Truth, Jordan Rubin discusses the rise in obesity among teenage girls in the 90's. "It turns out that it wasn't fat that was making them fat - it was eating foods with excess carbohydrates, especially processed foods. Cakes and cookies (especially the fat-free versions) seemed to be the culprit." Raw nuts, raw seeds, avocados and coconuts are healthy sources of fats.

Minerals - Only plants have the ability to convert dead, inorganic minerals from the soil to living organic minerals used by the animal kingdom. The animal kingdom cannot do this. Why do we think we can put dead substances into our living bodies and expect it to produce life? The majority of foods that Americans consume have not a trace of anything living by the time they reach our dinner table. The body uses minerals for most all life-maintaining functions. Lack of real food source minerals can result in a number of health problems, including tooth decay, fragile bones, mental fatigue and depression, liver ailments, digestive disorders, weakened eyesight, and many more. Dr. Robbins reminds us that it is "rare that one would ever suffer from a single mineral deficiency." The solution is not to treat the body with a single mineral, but instead to discern which whole foods are lacking in the diet.

Vitamins (Enzymes) - These are organic compounds that the body uses as catalysts to allow the life-maintaining chemical activities to take place. Vitamins occur naturally in all fruits and vegetables and are necessary for the normal functioning of the body. Raw, whole foods are the only true source of complete vitamins. According to Katy Chamberlin on the amazingdiscoveries.org post concerning refined grains, "over 20 vitamin and mineral elements are removed when whole wheat is converted into white flour, yet only four or five are replaced by enrichment. And these are supplied in an inferior synthetic form, which the body cannot use, and that does more harm than good." A real food diet will provide all the vitamins needed by the body.

Water - Water is used for every chemical or metabolic function in the body to maintain life. We can get water from the food we consume, the oxidation of food, and the intake of fluids directly. Plants contain an abundant amount of water. So with a naturally right diet, in other words a diet full of real foods, the need for the direct consumption of fluids is greatly reduced. But then again, its not like we are drinking our morning coffee or afternoon diet cola for the water.

Well, after looking at these six nutritional requirements, have you noticed a trend? Real foods come from the plant kingdom. Most real foods can be eaten in their raw state without any processing. Let me clarify. That means no microwaves, no chemical additives or preservatives, no added sugar, no refinement, no high fructose corn syrup, no long lists of unrecognizable ingredients. Just raw, real food. Lack of these real foods in our diet causes nutritional stress on the body, robbing it of energy, and therefore, health and vitality. "A diet of raw fruits, vegetables, sprouts, seeds and nuts will provide all of the nutrients that are needed for the body to function properly", says Dr. Robbins. If we want healthier families, we have to bring these REAL FOODS back into our homes!

Renal Diet Guidelines

There is no one specific "renal diet", only guidelines to help you control the levels of salts in your bloodstream through what you eat. The diet required for renal deficiency varies with each case, the severity of the malfunction, whether swelling is present, whether you are over-weight, what your blood electrolyte readings are, and whether you are a candidate for dialysis or not.

With renal failure, the salts in the bloodstream are completely thrown off balance. The aim of renal diet guidelines is to help control the build-up of waste products and fluid in your blood by placing less pressure on your kidneys.

Renal diet guidelines are built around blood test results and a normal healthy balanced diet. The idea is to limit the intake of salts that are too high. Fluids may also be restricted if your kidneys are unable to excrete sufficient water. Protein intake is limited so wastes like urea are kept at a minimum.

The salts that commonly need to be restricted are:

Sodium. Sodium can cause high blood pressure and fluid retention. Most renal diets use minimal salt in cooking, and stipulate, "No added salts". "Lo-salt" combinations are not suitable for salt replacement as they have high potassium levels, and should not be used. Processed foods, sausages, sauces, ketchup's and many canned foods should be avoided.

Phosphorus cannot be removed by dialysis, so it might become a problem. Levels are monitored, and kept under control by diet and sometimes medication. High phosphorus foods include dairy products, beans, peas, beer and cola drinks.

Potassium should only be restricted if the blood levels are high. Many healthy vegetables and fruits contain potassium. High potassium foods include apricots, orange juice, bananas, avocados, beets, spinach and many more.

Proteins are a necessary part of a healthy diet, but should only be eaten in small amounts. Proteins that should be restricted, include all meats, fish, eggs and dairy products.

Fluids might be restricted if water retention is present in the form of generalized swelling or fluid in the lungs. Fluids are often strictly controlled for patients on haemodialysis. Fluids include all beverages, soups, water and juices.

Carbohydrates are energy foods and should not be restricted unless you are a diabetic or overweight. Lastly, it might be advisable to take vitamin and antioxidant supplements to boost your immune system.

Following renal diet guidelines will help decrease the workload on damaged kidneys and slow down the loss of kidney function. The renal diet guidelines are intended to help keep kidney sufferers healthy and functional by eating to support and augment their treatment. It is very important to get specific advice from your doctor and dietitian at all times.

Kidney Foods Diet For Hemodialysis

Damage to our kidneys can either be temporary or permanent, and either way you most definitely do not want this to happen to your kidneys. Once our kidneys begin to fail, we experience a lot of symptoms that can be as subtle as a simple loss of appetite to even greater symptoms such as arrhythmias or even coma.

However, when you already have damaged kidneys and are undergoing hemodialysis there are still some kidney foods that you can take to better hasten the healing process of your kidneys. In choosing which food to include in your diet, you simply have to take note of certain nutrients that are essential for your speedy recovery. Below is a list of nutrients that one should increase or decrease when undergoing hemodialysis.

Calcium and phosphorous usually work in adjunct to each other, and they actually do more than just keeping our teeth and bones strong. A change in one of these two nutrients will also affect the other. Usually, once your kidneys fail, phosphorous tends to build up in the blood. Having high levels of phosphorous in the blood is never a good thing because it can lead to a lot of problems such as brittle bones, or even heart damage. So it is a good idea to decrease your phosphorous intake while also taking calcium implements just to prevent certain complications.

Sodium is also one nutrient that should be limited in a renal diet. Limiting sodium intake can help to control blood pressure and fluid build up, which are common signs of kidney failure. Sodium is commonly found in salt, so decrease intake of foods that are high in sodium such as processed foods, snack foods, and canned foods.

Usually when one is undergoing hemodialysis, one tends to lose a lot of proteins. As we all know, proteins are helpful in repairing tissues, fighting infection, and building muscles. So it is a good idea to increase your intake of food high in protein. Egg whites are a great source of proteins and they are much safer than meat.

These are only some of the nutrients that you should look for in kidney foods. Though it can be challenging to follow, keep in mind that well nourished patients actually recover faster and at the same time have fewer chances of getting infection.

Potassium Diet - A Low Potassium Diet For Kidney Disease

If you are someone that suffers from weakened or diseased kidneys, then you need to be very careful about the foods you eat. A good kidney Diet plan will help you to keep an eye on minerals like potassium and calcium that can easily start to build up in the body due to the kidneys being unable to rid the body of them in time. Getting too much potassium can lead to a problem called hyperkalemia, which involves having too high of a concentration of potassium in the blood. If you suffer from kidney problems, you will need to watch how much potassium you get each day to avoid this.

Normally, it is recommended people get around 4700 mg potassium each day. For those that are suffering form a chronic kidney disease that amount should be no more than 2700 mg. To stay within these boundaries, a good kidney Diet plan should consist of things like three servings of vegetables and three servings of fruits that are low in potassium each day, such as lettuce, cucumbers, and apples. Dairy is a good option because it is low in potassium and the calcium it has is easy for the body to absorb. Try to get one or two servings of dairy each day. This can include things like cheddar cheese and a small amount of margarine.

A good kidney Diet plan will usually contain between three and seven servings of meats that are low in potassium each day. Turkey breast is always a healthy choice, and you can have a hard boiled egg as well. When it comes to grains, between four and seven servings will be fine. Some good foods that fall into the grain category that are also low in potassium include white bread, English muffins, and non sweetened corn cereal.

A good low potassium diet can still involve you enjoying all or most of your favourite vegetables. The only recommendation is that you LEACH the vegetables before consumption. The process of leaching will help pull potassium out of some high-potassium vegetables. However, you should bear in mind that leaching will not pull out all of the potassium from your vegetables.

Once you get accustomed to a good Kidney Diet plan that is low in potassium you will see that it's not terribly challenging to follow. As long as you avoid the fruits like bananas and kiwis that are very high in potassium and make sure to drink enough fluids, you should be in good shape.

Renal Stones

Individuals with renal stones present with flank pain and hematuria with or without having fever. Based on the level of the rock and also the patient's underlying anatomy (e.g., if there is only an individual working kidney or significant preexisting renal illness), the presentation might be complicated by obstruction with decreased or absent urine production.

Even though a range of disorders may outcome in the improvement of renal stones, a minimum of 75% of renal stones contain calcium. Most instances of calcium stones are due to idiopathic hypercalciuria, with hyperuricosuria and hyperparathyroidism as other major causes. Uric acid stones are typically caused by hyperuricosuria, especially in individuals with a history of gout or excessive purine consumption (eg, a diet plan higher in organ meat products).

Defective amino acid transport, as occurs in cystinuria, can outcome in stone creation. Lastly, struvite stones, made up of magnesium, ammonium, and phosphate salts, are a outcome of chronic or recurrent urinary tract infection by urease-producing organisms (usually Proteus). Renal stones outcome from alterations in the solubility of various substances in urine, such that there is nucleation and precipitation of salts. A number of factors can tip the balance in favor of rock creation.

Dehydration favors rock formation, along with a high fluid intake to maintain a daily urine volume of a couple of L or a lot more seems to be defensive. The precise mechanism of this protection is unknown. Hypotheses include dilution of unfamiliar substances that predispose to stone formation and decreased transit time of Ca2+ through the nephron, minimizing the likelihood of precipitation.

A high-protein diet plan predisposes to rock formation in susceptible people. A dietary protein load causes transient metabolic acidosis and an elevated GFR. Even though serum Ca2+ is not detectably elevated, there is most likely a transient improve in calcium resorption from bone, an improve in glomerular calcium filtration, and inhibition of distal tubular calcium resorption. This effect appears to be greater in known stone-formers than in wholesome controls.

A high-Na+ diet plan predisposes to Ca2+ excretion and calcium oxalate rock formation, whereas a reduced dietary Na+ intake has the opposite effect. Furthermore, urinary Na+ excretion raises the saturation of monosodium urate, which can act as a nidus for Ca2+ crystallization. Despite the truth that most stones are calcium oxalate stones, oxalate concentration in the diet is generally as well low to assistance a recommendation to avoid oxalate to avoid stone creation.

Similarly, calcium restriction, formerly a main dietary recommendation to calcium rock formers, is beneficial only towards the subset of individuals whose hypercalciuria is diet plan dependent. In others, decreased nutritional calcium might actually improve oxalate absorption and predispose to rock creation.

A ⬚uantity of elements are defensive against rock creation.

In order of decreasing importance, fluids, citrate, magnesium, and nutritional fiber appear to use a defensive impact. Citrate might prevent rock formation by chelating calcium in solution and forming extremely soluble complexes in comparison with calcium oxalate and calcium phosphate.

Even though pharmacologic supplementation from the diet with potassium citrate has been shown to improve urinary citrate and pH and decrease the incidence of recurrent rock formation, the benefits of the naturally high-citrate diet plan have not been investigated. Nevertheless, some studies suggest that vegetarians use a lower incidence of stone formation.

Presumably, they avoid the stone-forming impact of high protein and Na+ within the diet plan, combined using the defensive effects of fiber along with other factors. Rock formation per se within the renal pelvis is painless until a fragment breaks off and travels down the ureter, precipitating ureteral colic. Hematuria and renal harm can occur in the absence of pain.

The discomfort associated with renal stones is due to distention from the ureter, renal pelvis, or renal capsule. The severity of discomfort is related towards the degree of distention that happens and thus is extremely severe in acute obstruction. Anuria and azotemia are suggestive of bilateral obstruction or unilateral obstruction of an individual working kidney.

The pain, hematuria, as well as ureteral obstruction caused by a renal stone are typically self-limited. For smaller stones, passage usually demands only fluids, bed rest, and analgesia. The major complications are (1) hydronephrosis and permanent renal harm as a result of total obstruction of the ureter, with resulting backup of urine and buildup of pressure; (a couple of) infection or abscess creation behind a partially or completely obstructing stone, which could rapidly destroy the involved kidney; (three) renal harm subsequent to repeated kidney stones; and (4) hypertension resulting from elevated renin production by the obstructed kidney.

The delicate diet of a renal patient

Our kidneys, like the lungs are paired organs that work equally to eliminate wastes in the body while removing excess water from the blood. Surprisingly, a human body could survive with one kidney alone and is able to live a normal life. No organ in the body could replace the function of the kidneys. There are certain instances that render the functions of both kidneys, making our bodies unable to process waste materials like urine. Kidney illnesses are characterized from mild to life-threatening problems. More often, people that suffer from kidney failures undergo treatment called hemodialysis were the blood is being filtered via a machine, removing wastes materials that is poisonous to the body and getting rid of excess fluids in the blood. Some only uses dialysis in short period of time until their kidneys are able to function, while others with complete kidney failure, the procedure are a lifetime process. People that undergo dialysis are required to follow a strict diet. Sad to say there are a lot restrictions regarding the diet of a renal patient.

Low sodium foods

A person who undergoes dialysis is not allowed to eat high sodium foods. Sodium attracts water like a magnet, since the function of the kidneys of a renal patient is low to none, excess fluids inside the body is very deadly. Medical experts and doctors are very strict regarding the diet of a renal patient; they know that one wrong move could be fatal.

Low potassium foods

Potassium like sodium also attracts fluid in our body. Although they could cancel each other out excess quantities to both fluids would be unhealthy to renal patient. Potassium rich foods are very abundant to the market. We all know that fruits are very beneficial to our health, however, there are certain types of fruits that is not appropriate to a renal patient. Mangos, avocados, watermelons and papaya are some of the potassium rich fruits, while apple and pineapple are allowed in the diet of a renal patient. Carrots, celery, cucumber, red pepper, and green pepper are low potassium vegetables are included to the diet of the dialysis patient.

Restrict fluids

A renal patient is required to monitor his or her fluid intake, excess fluids could cause damage to remaining healthy organs in the body. Soups and Oatmeal should be taken at a minimal manner.

The diet of a renal patient is very fragile. We must familiarize ourselves of the allowed and not allowed foods, if not their conditions could worsen. The key to any diet is balance; if we could attain that, our heath would be secured.

Diet For Kidney Failure - Are They Really Effective In Reducing The Progression Of Kidney Diseases?

As a nurse for many years now, a lot of people complain to me that their diet for kidney failure is so hard to follow. They tell me that this type of diet has too many restrictions and that it is so rigid and unforgiving.

My reply to the above statement is that maybe the asking patient didn't consider other possibilities of the diet? Or maybe he or she was not able to research enough to realize that this diet is in fact easy to follow.

Before I start talking about the diet for kidney failure, I will first talk a little about the kidney. The kidneys play key roles in body function, not only by filtering the blood and getting rid of waste products, but also by balancing levels of electrolytes in the body, controlling blood pressure, and stimulating the production of red blood cells.

Now, renal failure results when the kidneys cannot remove the body's metabolic wastes or perform their regulatory functions. The substances normally eliminated in the urine accumulate in the body fluids. As a result of this impaired renal excretion, there are electrolyte and acid-base disturbances.

Renal failure is a systemic disease and is final common pathway of many different kidney and urinary tract diseases. Each year, the number of deaths from irreversible renal failure increases.

Kidney disease diet is an important consideration for those with impaired kidney function. Consultation with a dietitian may be helpful to understand what foods may or may not be appropriate. Various kidney disease recipes are available in the market right now.

Since the kidneys cannot easily remove excess water, salt, or potassium, they may need to be consumed in limited quantities. Foods high in potassium include bananas, apricots, and salt substitutes.

Phosphorus is a forgotten chemical that is associated with calcium metabolism and may be elevated in kidney failure. Too much phosphorus can leech calcium from the bones and cause osteoporosis and fractures. Foods with high phosphorus content include milk, cheese, nuts, and cola drinks.

This diet is usually done with other treatments for kidney failure. The two major treatments for kidney failure are dialysis and transplantation. The former has two kinds of procedures-hemodialysis (accessed via IV route) and peritoneal dialysis (done via the abdomen). The latter, on the other hand, involves a more complex pre-operation.

With a research based diet for kidney failure, renal recovery is almost guaranteed. It is, however, important to be started as immediately as possible to prevent long term damage.

What you need to know about chronic renal failure

Chronic Renal Failure will usually happen in stages and not all at once. The frequent causes of CRF are from:

1. Uncontrolled diabetes type 1 and type 2

2. Uncontrolled Hypertension

3. Chronic Urinary Tract Infections

4. Polycystic Kidney Disease

5. Glomerulonephritis is a chronic kidney destructive problem that gradually tears away at the glomeruli in the kidney.

When you are having chronic renal faliure, your kidneys are slowly dying until your kidneys reach end-stage-renal failure. In the earliest stages of chronic renal failure, there will hardly be any symptoms that are noticed. As it continues to progress however, symptoms will slowly appear. The symptoms that are the most common as chronic renal failure progresses are:

1. Hiccups

2. Tiredness

3. Malaise (Unwell feeling)

4. Sick to your stomach and throwing up meals a lot

5. Weight loss that is unexplainable

6. Bad headache pain

7. Intensive itching that will drive you crazy

8. Hypertension

9. There is a high amount of protein in the urine

As chronic renal failure goes on, there will be some very debilitating symptoms that will continue. These prominent symptoms are those like:

1. You are vomiting up blood

2. Not producing very much if any urine, and what little produced is blood, (hematuria)

3. Not feeling anything, (the sensory nerves being affected)

4. Leg cramps

5. Urea on the skin and breath which is in the form of a chalky type of white substance

When urea is appearing on the skin, it means uremia, which is a fancy medical term for kidney failure.

Blood tests in chronic renal failure in the first stages will not be that bad. But as this process goes on, the blood tests will show some very poor results.

Creatnine blood levels will rise, and the glomerular filtration rate (gfr) will steadily drop. This is telling you that your kidneys want to perform less and less.

BUN, which is Blood Urea Nitrogen tells whether or not the urea is being processed well by the kidneys or not. A level that is starting to rise above 39 or more means trouble.

A blood test for potassium is going to be high, reflecting that the kidneys are not processing your potassium and letting it become toxic to you in your blood.

Sodium levels may also be out of sight in the bloodstream. This is another key factor that kidneys are not letting go of sodium properly, and therefore, this too builds up in the blood.

Calcium levels will be high too since kidneys will not process calcium either due to the fact that nephrons are being destroyed.

The whole goal of treating chronic renal failure is to slow down the process so that you can stay clear of actual kidney failure altogether for as long as possible.

Diuretics will be part of your care regime as well as potassium binders which hold back the potassium levels from going too high. The diuretic medications will get rid of excess water as long as you are still making urine. Calcium binders will be added as well since calcium is another substance that is going to build up extremely high from the kidneys failing to process it in the blood.

A special diet is a must for those with advanced stages of chronic renal failure. Part of the diet is fluid restrictions since urine production gradually declines. Your intake of sodium, potassium, and calcium will be limited to certain amounts daily. A specialized dietitian will need to sit down with you to work out your daily dietary plans according to your kidney doctor's recommendations.

Atural Treatment For Renal Calculi

If you are suffering from kidney stones there are a number of treatment for renal calculi options that are available to you. Kidney stones are crystalline materials formed in the kidney and there are a number of risk factors associated with the development of renal calculi.

Chronically high amounts of uric acid in the blood can cause the formation of kidney stones as can decreases in the amount of urine and dehydration. Having certain health conditions such as gout, urinary tract infection, hypertension and diabetes can increase the risk of urate stones. Having a family history of renal calculi can also put you at greater risk of developing kidney stones.

Symptoms and Diagnoses

Symptoms of renal calculi include difficulty urinating, blood in the urine and excruciating pain in the lower back, side, abdomen and groin. If you have any of these symptoms you should immediately seek treatment for renal calculi. The usual test for diagnosing kidney stones is a helical CT scan that will detect the presence of renal calculi in the urinal tract. For pregnant women who cannot be exposed to radiation, an ultrasound examination may be performed.

Most renal stones will pass through the urinary tract on their own within two days, so long as the patient takes sufficient fluids. If the pain of the passage is too intense, doctors may prescribe pain killers to ease the suffering. If the renal stones are too large to pass through the urinary tract, surgery may be prescribed as a treatment for renal calculi.

Recently, extracorporeal shock wave therapy (ESWT) was developed to remove kidney stones without the need for surgery. ESWT uses sound waves precisely aimed at the kidney stone that causes it to dissolve into smaller pieces that can easily be passed through the urinary tract or dissolve into the body.

Natural Noninvasive Treatments

There are a number of natural treatment for renal calculi options available to help those with a genetic propensity towards kidney stones from developing them. These include:

Diet modification that includes increasing the amount of water intake to at least 50% of a person's body weight as expressed in ounces (i.e. if you weigh 180 pounds you should drink at least 90 oz of water daily) as well as a diet rich in fresh fruits and vegetables and low in foods that are rich in purine.

Avoiding alcoholic beverages since they promote the buildup of uric acid, processed sugars, fish such as salmon and sardines and refined wheat products such as white bread, cookies and other pastries.

Taking magnesium supplements, since the lack of magnesium in the system has been linked to the formation of kidney stones.

Aerobic exercise is good to improve the blood flow and sweating is an effective way to excrete excess minerals and toxins out from the body which can help to reduce the burden on the kidneys.

Know about the different stages of renal failure

Many illnesses are classified into numerous stages based on their severity and the negative effects they cause on the patient's body. In the same way, renal failure is also classified into 5 main stages, which are based on the GFR or glomerular filtration rate. The various stages in this ailment are:

• Stage 1

A GFR of 90 or more is identified under this category. The symptoms in stage 1 and 2 are blood pressure and creatinine that are higher than the normal level; traces of protein or blood found in urine; indications are found to point towards genetic factors that trigger this ailment. The treatment at this stage is generally aimed at preventing heart disease and reducing the risk of diabetes.

• Stage 2

When compared to the previous stage, the renal system starts functioning slower, indicating that things are taking a turn for the worse. Similar to stage 1, the observation of the various risk factors like blood pressure is followed diligently in this stage too. Here, the GFR hovers between 60 and 89.

• Stage 3

In some cases, this stage is further divided into 2 parts as 3A and 3B, wherein the GFR is 45-59 and 30-44 respectively. But unfortunately, your health starts deteriorating further giving way to problems like bone wear and tear and anemia. There may be a considerable loss of red blood cells due to a malfunctioning renal system. So, it is important to consult a registered medical practitioner to get treatment for these complications first so that they do not grow further and play spoilsport on your health.

• Stage 4

Stage 4 should give you a red signal that it is time for some serious action to save the renal system for the GFR is found at very low levels, i.e. 15-29 only. In medical terms, this acts as a pointer towards the fact that the renal system is heading towards a grinding halt as it is severely affected by now. In many cases, the patients are prescribed a suitable form of dialysis, that is, either peritoneal dialysis or hemodialysis. In some cases, in this stage, your medical practitioner will suggest opting for long-term dialysis or renal transplant as found suitable for you.

• Stage 5

This is the most dangerous stage in renal failure since the GFR is below 15. This means your renal system is functioning at a very worrisome level. There are many symptoms like nausea, fatigue, frequent headaches, change in skin color, etc. This stage can be life-threatening in some cases if there are other complications acting as triggering factors. Dialysis or transplant has to be carried out earnestly and carefully too.

So, you now have a fairly good idea about the various stages in renal failure and how to treat them effectively. In all these stages, it is important to adhere to the prescribed diet and medication schedules.

Diet and exercise help reduce risk of kidney failure

Kidney failure has become a relatively common medical condition in the United States due to a rise in the prevalence of diet and exercise related diseases over the past several years. Generally, people spend very little time considering the important role that the kidneys play and the actions that can be taken to reduce the risk of kidney damage. Awareness of what the kidneys do and how they can be harmed tends to increase dramatically once someone has developed end stage renal disease and is faced with the need for dialysis or a kidney transplant. Increasing public awareness through education may help reduce the trend towards a greater dependence on long-term treatments like dialysis.

The kidneys are critical to the maintenance of a healthy balance of fluid and nutrients in the body. The bloodstream, within the average human, passes through the kidneys many times each day carrying with it wastes that have the potential of causing serious harm to the body if they are not excreted. As the blood passes through the kidneys, excess water and waste are allowed to leave while useful nutrients are reabsorbed into the blood. When the kidneys are damaged by diseases, they can no longer maintain a healthy balance and the body begins to deteriorate. Dialysis is often required to restore a part of the filtration process that would normally be performed by the kidneys.

Diabetes is the most common cause of kidney failure in the United States today. This condition can be divided into two groups depending on the way in which it occurs. Type 1 Diabetes results when the immune system attacks the insulin producing cells of the pancreas causing them to stop producing insulin. Type 2 Diabetes results when the body's cells become unresponsive to the insulin that is being produced by the pancreas. In both cases, a harmful level of sugar is allowed to circulate through the blood causing damage to many different organs. Poorly controlled diabetes can result in end stage renal disease and possibly even a kidney transplant.

It is important for dialysis technicians and other clinical staff to understand the importance of diabetes in kidney failure so that they can educate patients on what can be done to manage the disease. Patients are often unfamiliar with how the kidneys work and how they can be damaged. Since dialysis technicians spend so much time with patients, they are in an excellent position to inform patients about many different aspects of their illness. Many patients are more willing to cooperate with treatment and comply with the prescribed therapy once they understand what is happening in their body.

High blood pressure is another major cause of kidney failure in the United States. There are many different reasons for why an individual might develop high blood pressure, but poor diet and lack of exercise are two of the most common. The consumption of foods high in salt along with a sedentary lifestyle in the United States has led to large numbers of people who are well above their healthy body weight and who suffer from numerous diet and exercise related illnesses. Medical professionals who are aware of this fact are in a better position to inform patients about changes that they can make in their life that can reduce the risk of requiring long-term care. In addition, individuals who have high blood pressure can be placed on medications that have been developed to help reduce the blood pressure.

The combined effect of a healthy diet, regular exercise, and medications can help patients avoid the complications of end stage renal disease so that they can live a happier and healthier life. While no amount of treatment can fully replace the damage that is caused by diabetes and high blood pressure, many patients find that they are able to go on living a reasonably healthy life. Dialysis patients also become an important resource for educating others about the potential negative consequences of a poor diet and a lack of exercise. Through the combined efforts of patients and healthcare professionals, it is believed that future cases of kidney failure can be prevented.

Chronic Renal Failure - Specialized Ayurvedic Treatment

Chronic kidney disease is defined as kidney damage or a decreased kidney glomerular filtration rate of less than 60, for 3 months or more, irrespective of the cause. This results in a progressive decline in kidney function, resulting in accumulation of toxic waste products, excess water and salts, increased blood pressure, anemia and many other complex symptoms. Chronic renal failure is divided into Stages I - V, out of which the first three stages are asymptomatic, and usually discovered incidentally, while doing routine blood tests.

The management of chronic renal failure consists of treatment of the underlying cause if possible, aggressive treatment of high blood pressure and other symptoms, liquid and diet control, cessation of smoking, and finally, with end-stage disease, resorting to dialysis or a kidney transplant.

The Ayurvedic treatment of chronic renal failure is based on three principles:

(i)   treating the damaged kidneys
(ii)   reating the body tissues (dhatus) which make up the kidneys and
(iii)   treating the known cause.

The damage done to the kidneys can be repaired using medicines like Punarnavadi Guggulu, Gokshuradi Guggulu, Gomutra Haritaki, Chandraprabha Vati and Punarnavadi Qadha (decoction). Herbal medicines useful in this condition are: Punarnava (Boerhaavia diffusa), Gokshur (Tribulus terrestris), Haritaki (Terminalia chebula), Neem (Azadirachta indica), Daruharidra (Berberis aristata) and Patol (Tricosanthe dioica).

According to Ayurveda, the kidneys are made up of the "Rakta" and "Meda" dhatus. Treating these two dhatus is also an effective way to treat the kidneys. Medicines used are: Patol, Saariva, Patha (Cissampelos pareira), Musta (Cyperus rotundus), Kutki (Picrorrhiza kurroa),

Chirayta (Swertia chirata), Guduchi (Tinospora cordifolia), Chandan (Santalum album) and Shunthi (Zinziber officinalis).

Lastly, the known cause of chronic renal failure is treated using medicines which also act upon the kidneys. Vascular (related to the blood vessels) diseases like renal artery stenosis and inflammation of the artery walls(vasculitis) can be treated using medicines like Arogya Vardhini, Tapyadi Loha, Mahamanjishthadi Qadha, Kamdudha Vati, Manjishtha (Rubia cordifolia), Bhrungraj (Eclipta alba), Saariva, Kutki and Sarpagandha (Rauwolfia serpentina). Primary glomerular diseases like membranous nephropathy and glomerlonephritis can be treated using Punarnava, Gokshur, Saariva and Manjishtha. Secondary glomerular disease resulting from diabetes, systemic lupus erythematosus, rheumatoid arthritis etc. can be treated accordingly, using the medicines appropriate for those diseases. Similarly, suitable Ayurvedic medicines can be given for other causes like polycystic kidneys, prostate enlargement and neurogenic bladder.

The advantage of using Ayurvedic medicines in chronic renal failure is that in most patients, the kidney damage can be either partly or fully reversed, the frequency of dialysis can be reduced, and the increased risk of death from cardiovascular diseases can be significantly reduced. Thus, Ayurvedic medicines have the potential for an important therapeutic contribution in all the stages of this condition.

For patients with chronic renal failure intending to take Ayurvedic treatment (or for that matter, any alternative treatment), the following points should be kept in mind: (i) all patients should be under the regular supervision and treatment of a ⬚ualified and experienced Urologist (ii) Ayurvedic medicines should be taken in the form of additional treatment, and should not replace other, regular treatment or dialysis and (iii) the attending Urologist should be informed of the decision to start Ayurvedic treatment.

High protein diets - myths, half-truths and outright lies

Without ⬚uestion, protein is the king of all nutrients. It provides the building blocks for enzymes and hormones, enables nerve and brain cells to effectively communicate with one another, and fosters the repair and growth of muscle tissue. Every cell in your body contains protein; life could not go on without it.

The consumption of protein, however, is perhaps the most controversial of all nutritional topics. Unfortunately, many nutrition professionals have not kept abreast of recent research and continue to espouse outmoded theories on the subject. This has led to a host of myths that, in turn, have been taken as gospel by the general public. The following are some of the more common misconceptions about dietary protein intake:

Myth: High protein diets make you fat.

Fact: There is no doubt that eating too much protein will pack on the pounds-but so will eating too many calories from carbs or fat! Weight gain is governed by the law of thermodynamics: if you consume more calories than you expend, you'll gain weight. Conse🞆uently, it's not protein per se that causes weight gain; it's an over consumption of calories. No matter what you eat, if you consume too much of it, you'll ultimately end up getting fat.

In actuality, if you were to eat a meal containing only protein, carbs, or fat, the protein meal would cause the least amount of weight gain. You see, a large percentage of calories from protein are burned off in the digestion process. This is called the thermic effect of food. Of all the macronutrients, protein has the highest thermic effect, burning off approximately 25 percent of protein of the calories consumed . In comparison, only 15 percent of the calories from carbs are burned off in digestion; fat has virtually no thermic effect whatsoever . Thus, all other things being equal, a high protein diet would be less likely to cause fat deposition than either a high carb or high fat diet.

Moreover, unlike carbs, protein doesn't stimulate a significant insulin response. Insulin is a storage hormone. While its primary purpose is to neutralize blood sugar, it also is responsible for shuttling fat into adipocytes (fat cells). When carbohydrates are ingested, the pancreas secretes insulin to clear blood sugar from the circulatory system. Depending on the quantities and types of carbs consumed, insulin levels can fluctuate wildly, heightening the possibility of fat storage. Since protein's effect on insulin secretion is negligible, the potential for fat storage is diminished

What's more, the consumption of protein tends to increase the production of glucagon, a hormone that opposes the effect of insulin. Since a primary function of glucagon is to signal the body to burn fat for fuel, fat loss, rather than fat gain, tends to be promoted.

Myth: High protein diets are damaging to your kidneys.

Fact: The metabolism of protein entails a complex sequence of events in order for proper assimilation to take place. During digestion, protein is broken down into its component parts, the amino acids (via a process called deamination). A byproduct of this occurrence is the production of ammonia, a toxic substance, in the body. Ammonia, in turn, is rapidly converted into the relatively non-toxic substance urea, which is then transported to the kidneys for excretion.

In theory, a large build-up of urea can overtax the kidneys, impairing their ability to carry out vital functions. This has been supported by studies on people with existing renal disease. It has been well documented that a high protein diet exacerbates uremia (kidney failure) in those on dialysis (i.e. the artificial kidney machine), while a low protein diet helps to alleviate the condition . Proteinuria and other complications also have been observed in this population .

However, there is no evidence that a diet high in protein has any detrimental effects on those with normal renal function. Healthy kidneys are readily able to filter out urea; any excess is simply expelled in the urine. Consider the fact that, over the past century, millions of athletes have consumed large quantities of protein without incident. Surely, if high protein diets caused kidney disease, these athletes would be all on dialysis by now. Yet, in otherwise healthy individuals, not one peer-reviewed journal has documented any renal abnormalities due to an increased intake of protein.

As an aside, it is beneficial to drink ample amounts of fluids when consuming a high protein diet. This helps to flush your system and facilitates the excretion of urea from the body. For best results, a daily intake of at least a gallon of water is recommended, drinking small amounts throughout the day.

Myth: High protein diets result in an inordinate intake of unhealthy saturated fat.

Fact: The majority of Americans get their protein from red meat and dairy products-foods that have a high percentage of saturated fat. High fat protein sources such as bacon, T-bone steaks, hard cheeses, and whole milk are staples of the American diet. What's more, ketogenic "diet gurus" like Dr. Robert Atkins encourage the consumption of these products, touting them as viable dietary options . Accordingly, high-protein diets have become synonymous with the intake artery-clogging fats.

However, there is no reason that a high protein intake must be derived from cholesterol-laden foods. There are many protein sources that contain little, if any, saturated fat. Skinless chicken breasts, egg whites, and legumes are all excellent, low-fat protein choices. By simply choosing the "right" foods, a high protein diet can be maintained with minimal effect on fat consumption.

In addition, it is important to realize that certain fats, specifically the unsaturated, Omega fatty acids, are actually beneficial to your well being, aiding in the absorption of fat-soluble vitamins and facilitating the production of various hormones, cell membranes and prostaglandins. These "essential" fats cannot be manufactured by the body and hence must be obtained through nutritional means. Cold water fish (such as salmon, mackerel and trout), tofu and peanut butter are protein-based foods that also are terrific sources of essential fats. Their consumption has been shown to have a positive impact on cardiovascular health and reduces the risk of several types of cancers.

Myth: High protein diets are unnecessary for athletes.

Fact: If you believe the United States Department of Agriculture (USDA), there is no difference in protein reᐧuirements between athletes and couch potatoes. This is reflected in the RDA for protein, which is the same for all individuals regardless of their activity levels.

However, contrary to the USDA position, studies have shown that athletes do indeed reᐧuire more protein than sedentary individuals . When you exercise, protein stores are broken down and used for fuel (via a process called gluconeogenesis). The branched chain amino acids (BCAAs), in particular, are preferentially mobilized as an energy source during intense training, as are alanine and glutamine. It has been shown that when athletes consume a low protein diet (equivalent to the RDA for protein), there is decreased whole body protein synthesis, indicating a catabolism of muscle tissue.

On the other hand, it is imprudent to ingest enormous ⸮uantities of protein in hopes that it will improve athletic performance. Bodybuilders often subscribe to this "more is better" philosophy and gorge themselves with protein-rich foods and supplements (one popular bodybuilder claims to ingest as much as 1000 grams of protein a day!). Unfortunately, the body only has the capacity to utilize a limited amount of protein. Once the saturation point is reached, additional protein is of no use to the body and is either used as energy or converted into triglycerides and stored as fat. In general, optimal protein synthesis can be achieved by consuming one gram of protein per pound of bodyweight. Thus, for maximizing strength and performance, a 150-pound person should consume approximately 150 grams of protein per day.

It also is important to realize that, by itself, protein has no effect on muscular gains. Contrary to claims made by various supplement manufacturers, protein powders aren't magic formulas for building muscle. You can't expect to simply consume a protein drink, sit back, and watch your muscles grow. This might make good ad copy, but it doesn't translate into reality. Only through intense strength training can protein be utilized for muscular repair and promote the development of lean muscle tissue.

What Everyone Should Know About Feline Chronic Renal Failure

Chronic Renal Failure or CRF is one of the most common age related illnesses in cats today. Chronic and progressive kidney failure is typically related to age, other illnesses and environment. Diet can play a part. CRF is always terminal, but with management of the disease, cats can live a quality life for many years after diagnosis.

The most obvious sign of CRF in a cat is excessive thirst, although there may be other symptoms, such as nausea, weight loss, constipation and a generally poor hair coat. Laboratory testing is required to make a definitive diagnosis. Lab results will also give the veterinarian a sense of how advanced the CRF is.

Diet and intravenous fluids are the most common therapies for cats with CRF. Dietary management means feeding a diet lower in protein, salt and phosphorous. Reducing these things will help the kidneys function better. A lower protein diet takes some of the burden off the kidneys for filtering waste, as protein molecules tend to be larger and create a heavier burden on the kidney. The kidneys are involved in electrolyte balance so the lower sodium and lower phosphorus allows the kidneys to maintain this balance more easily.

Intravenous fluid therapy helps keep the cat hydrated. Subcutaneous fluids can be administered at home by the owner and are often well tolerated by the cat. Being well hydrated allows the cat a general sense of well being. The fluids also flush the kidneys, ridding the body of built up toxins.

There are alternative healthcare treatments that may be helpful to a cat with CRF. There are many ⊡ualified holistic veterinarians who will be happy to consult with owners of CRF cats. Their specialized knowledge can guide owners towards the therapies that are best suited to their cat's health needs and temperament.

While many herbal remedies may be available over the counter and it is tempting to take the word of a trusted friend, it is not advisable to do so. Herbal remedies are a powerful medication and cats can react very strongly. Dosages and treatments should never be guessed at, but should be prescribed by a qualified veterinarian.

While CRF is considered a terminal disease, life can be considered terminal. It's hard to hear that your cat's days are numbered, but depending upon the severity of the disease, they may have many good years ahead of them. Managing CRF is less difficult than it sounds and the cat's life doesn't have to completely change. As knowledge and understanding of this disease progress, more and more cats are living longer and longer with their illness.

Our Menus

Now we have gathered seven daily menus for you. We have carefully prepared these menus to incorporate several recipes from this cookbook. Each menu in this book contains approximately 2000 calories, 70 grams of protein, 2 grams of sodium, 2 grams of potassium and 1 gram of phosphorus per day.

Day 1
• Breakfast
Take 3 Pepper Quiche, Two servings Pear half cup, Milk half cup
• Lunch
Cream of Crab Soup, Two slices of Sandwich: Garlic Bread, Two ounces of Roasted Beef One small Apple
• Dinner
• Take Turkey Fajitas. Two Avocado ¼, One cup of Strawberry Ice Cream

Day 2

• Breakfast

Fruit & Oat Pancakes, Two Margarine, Two teaspoons of Syrup, Two tablespoons of Cran Apple Juice 1/2 cup

• Lunch

Chili Con Carne, One cup of Corn Tortillas, One cup (6 inch) of Lemonade

• Dinner

Scampi Linguini, One cup of Carrots juice, One slice of Garlic Bread, Half cup Chocolate-Lover's Mousse.

Day 3

• Breakfast

One cup of Cream of Wheat, One slice of Zucchini Bread, One cup Cranberry Juice Cocktail, 2 teaspoons Margarine, Two teaspoons of Sugar, Half cup of Milk

• Lunch

Two cups of Niçoise, Pasta Salad, One Dinner Roll, Two teaspoons of Margarine, Half cup of Hot Fruit Compote

• Dinner

Three ounces of Meat Loaf, Broccoli-Cauliflower and Carrot Bake, Orzo Pasta, One slice of French Bread, Two teaspoons of Margarine, Half cup of Peaches.

Day 4

• Breakfast

Two slices Poached Eggs (Two) Toast, Two teaspoons of Margarine, Grapes, One cup of small Cranberry (Fifteen pieces) Juice Cocktail

• Lunch

Eat just two slices of Salt Free Pizza, Lettuce Salad (Half cup Sliced Cucumber, Two Teaspoon of Poppy Seed Dressing, and one small Orange

• Dinner

One cup of Sweet and Sour Chicken, Half cup of Egg Fried Rice, Three Plum one medium

Chinese Almond Cookies

Day 5

• Breakfast

Two slices of French toast, Two teaspoons of Margarine, Two tablespoons of Syrup, Half cup of Orange Juice

• Lunch

One and half cups Lemon Curry Chicken Salad, One Raspberry Streusel Muffin, Two teaspoon of Margarine, One cup of Pine-Apple Fruit Whip

• Dinner

One Festive Cajun Pork Chop, Half cup of Cranberry Stuffing, Half cup of Peas, One Dinner Roll, Two teaspoons of Margarine

Day 6

• Breakfast

Two Scrambled Eggs, One English Muffin, Two teaspoons of Margarine, One tablespoon of Jelly, Half cup of Peach Nectar

• Lunch

One cup of Cream of Corn Soup, Hamburger (Three ounces of Hamburger Patty, One Hamburger Bun, Two teaspoons of Mayonnaise, Half cup of Fruit Cocktail

• Dinner

Three ounces of Herb Topped Fish, Half cup of Barley-Rice Pilaf, Half cup of Steamed Green Beans, One Dinner Roll, Two teaspoons of Margarine

Day 7
• Breakfast
Two o Country Biscuits and with 1/3 cup of gravy, One cup of Strawberries
• Lunch
Half Grilled Chicken Sesame, Half cup of chicken breast Cottage Cheese Salad, Half slices of medium Tomato, Frosted Lemon Cookies

• Dinner

Two ounces of Onion Smothered Steak, Half cup of Moroccan Couscous, Half cup of Sunshine Carrots, One Dinner Roll, Two teaspoons of Margarine, 2/3 cup of Red Hot Jello Salad.

Appetizers And Snacks

Renal job

Chili wheat delight

Ingredients:

- Half cup of margarine
- One tablespoon chili powder
- Half teaspoon of ground cumin
- Half teaspoon of garlic powder
- Grace the dish with Dash cayenne pepper
- Four cups (spoon size) shredded wheat

Serving mode: You should serve half Cup per Serving

Directions: Heat oven to 300°F beforehand. Then you can melt your margarine in a 10 x 15 inch baking pan. Then you can stir in the spices. You can then add your cereal and stir properly so the mixture can coat evenly. Put it in the oven and then you bake for Fifteen minutes or until it becomes crispy. You can then store in a well-covered clean container.

Nutritional Facts

Nutrients				Renal and Renal Diabetic Exchanges
Calories	184	Sodium	107	One Starch
Carbohydrates	16	Potassium	104	One Low Potassium
Protein	3	Phosphorus	82	Vegetable
Fat	12			Two Fat

Eggnog delight

Ingredients:
- Half cup of margarine
- One tablespoon chili powder
- Half teaspoon of ground cumin
- Half teaspoon of garlic powder
- Grace the dish with Dash cayenne pepper
- Four cups (spoon size) shredded wheat

Serving mode: You should serve half Cup per Serving

Directions: Heat oven to 300°F beforehand. Then you can melt your margarine in a 10 x 15 inch baking pan. Then you can stir in the spices. You can then add your cereal and stir properly so the mixture can coat evenly. Put it in the oven and then you bake for Fifteen minutes or until it becomes crispy. You can then store in a well-covered clean container.

Nutrient	Renal and Renal Diabetic Exchanges
• Calories 134	1 Milk
• Carbohydrates 13	1 Fat
• Protein 3	
• Fat 8	

Onion delight chips

Ingredients:

- Two to Three and half oz of plain bagels
- Two tablespoons margarine melted
- Half teaspoon onion powder

Serving mode: Eight Chips per Serving

Directions:

- You are to cut each bagel into half vertically, making use of an electric knife.
- Place one bagel half, cut up side down, it should be on a flat surface; then you cut it vertically into 8 slices.
- Repeat the same procedure with the bagel halves remaining. Place the sliced bagels on a baking sheet. Mix margarine with onion powder and then brush it over the bagels.
- Bake the bagels at 325°F for up to 20 minutes or better still until it turns golden and crisp. Then you can remove them from pan; and allow to cool completely.

Store the ready to eat delicious Onion delight Chios in an airtight container.

Nutrients   Renal and Renal Diabetic Exchanges

- Calories 128   1 Starch
- Carbohydrates 16   1 Fat
- Protein 3
- Fat 6
- Sodium 208
- Potassium 24
- Phosphorus 24

Delicious egg rolls

Ingredients:

- One lb of diced cooked chicken
- Half lb of bean sprouts
- Half lb of shredded cabbage
- One medium (one cup) of chopped onion
- Two tablespoons of vegetable oil
- One tablespoon low sodium soy sauce
- One clove of garlic, minced
- One package "20" egg roll wrappers
- Vegetable oil for frying

Serving mode: One Egg Roll per Serving

Directions:

- You are to mix all ingredients except the wrappers and vegetable oil for frying together in a bowl. Then you let it marinate for about30 minutes.
- The next thing to do is to divide the filling among the wrappers and carefully fold as been directed on wrapper package instructions.
- Heat the oil up to 350°F beforehand.
- Fry your delicious egg rolls in hot vegetable oil until it turns golden brown.
- You are to now drain on paper towels.

Nutrients	Renal and Renal Diabetic Exchanges
• Calories 168	1 Starch
• Carbohydrates 15	1 Meat
• Protein 9	1 Fat
• Fat 8	
• Sodium 152	
• Potassium 114	
• Phosphorus 57	

Parmesan cheese spray

Ingredients:

• One to Three-oz of package cream cheese

• Four tablespoons of margarine (softened)

• 1/4 teaspoon of garlic powder

• Two tablespoons of grated Parmesan cheese

• One tablespoon of dry white wine

• One tablespoon of minced parsley

• A Sprinkle of thyme

• A Sprinkle of marjoram

Serving mode: Two tablespoons Per Serving is required

Directions: You are to mix all the ingredients very well until they blend very well. And then you chill for at least four hours. One of the good things about this delicacy is that you can serve with melba toast, unsalted crackers or better still as a stuffing for celery.

Nutrients	Renal and Renal Diabetic Exchanges
• Calories 109	Meat 1/3
• Carbohydrates 1	Fat 2
• Protein 2	
• Fat 11	
• Sodium 115	
• Potassium 24	
• Phosphorus 25	

Polynesian Kabobs Turkey
Ingredients:

• One lb of ground raw turkey
• 1/3 cup of unsalted crackers, (It has to be crushed five crackers)
• One egg or 1/4 cup of li?uid egg substitute
• 1/4 cup of chopped onion

- One teaspoon of ground ginger
- One clove garlic (crushed)
- One to Twenty-oz of canned pineapple chunks of its juice, properly reserved of up to 1/3 cup juice
- Add one large red pepper, then you cut it into twenty two pieces
- One large green pepper (Then cut into twenty three pieces)
- 1/3 cup of your reserved pineapple juice
- Two tablespoons of margarine (Make sure it's melted)
- Two tablespoons of orange marmalade
- One and half teaspoons of freshly ground ginger

Serving mode: One Skewer Per Serving

Directions:

- Get a medium bowl, and then mix it first with the six ingredients. Then you can shape them into 30 meat balls.
- Try to arrange them on 15 to 8-inch wooden board with your pineapple chunks and pepper pieces on it.
- After all that you can now place them on a broiler pan.
- Get a small bowl, and then stir the pineapple juice with margarine, marmalade and ginger very well until they blend pretty well.
- Brush them with kabobs.
- Then you can boil four inches from a heat source for twenty minutes, turning them once and carefully basting with sauce.

Nutrients   Renal and Renal

		Diabetic Exchanges
• Calories	95	One meat
• Carbohydrates	9	One low potassium
• Protein	8	
• Fat	3	Vegetable
• Sodium	49	
• Potassium	187	
• Phosphorus	72	

Popcorn delight

Ingredients:

- Two cups of graham cracker cereal
- Two cups of sweetened wheat puff cereal
- Eight cups of your fresh popped popcorn (unsalted)

Serving mode: One and half Cups Per Serving
Directions:
- Mix your cereals and popcorn in a microwavable bowl. Turn your Microwave on high for about one and half minutes or until it gets hot.
- Leave it for at least for five minutes.
- Let it break into pieces.

- Place in an oven, put your mixture into a metal pan and bake with temperature at 350°F for at least six minutes.
- Then you finally allow to cool for at least five minutes and until it breaks into pieces.

Nutrient			Renal and Renal Diabetic Exchanges
• Calories	122		One Starch
• Carbohydrates	20		One Fat
• Protein	2		
• Fat	4		
• Sodium	104		
• Phosphorus	46		
• Potassium	71		

Snacky mix

Ingredients:
- One cup of rice cereal box
- One cup of corn cereal box
- One cup of unsalted tiny pretzel mix
- Three cups of unsalted popped popcorn
- 1/3 cup of margarine (melted)
- Half teaspoon of garlic powder
- Half teaspoon of onion powder

• One tablespoon of Parmesan cheese
Serving mode: Six cups/ One cup Per Serving
Directions:
• Mix sugar, vinegar, lime juice, Dijon mustard, pepper and garlic powder in a sauce pan.
• Bring together and boil.
• Lower the heat and simmer, and then leave it uncovered for three minutes
• Mix the vinegar mixture and pineapple together in a bowl and mix them very well.
• And then you can serve warm with toothpicks

Nutrients		Renal and Renal Diabetic Exchanges
• Calories	47	One Low Potassium Fruit
• Carbohydrates	12	
• Protein	0	
• Fat	0	
• Sodium	4	
• Phosphorus	67	
• Potassium	4	

Spicy sweet meatballs

Ingredients:

• Use vegetable cooking spray
• 1/4 cup chopped onion

- One lb of lean ground chuck
- 1/3 cup of fine dry bread crumbs
- 1/4 cup of chopped very fresh parsley
- 1/8 teaspoon of nutmeg
- 1/4 cup of liquid non-dairy creamer
- One egg white, break and beat it
- Half cup cranberries, finely chopped
- Two teaspoons of dry mustard
- 1/8 teaspoon of cayenne pepper
- Half cup of grape jelly
- One teaspoon of lemon juice

Serving mode: Two Meatballs per Serving

Directions:
- You are to rub or coat a small sauce pan with cooking spray; you are to heat on medium heat source.
- You can then add onion and sauté until it becomes tender.
- Mix onion with the next six ingredients all in a bowl.
- You can then shape it into Thirty six to One-inch meat-balls.
- Then you can place meatballs on the baking sheet that has been coated with cooking spray.
- You are to bake at 375°F for about Eighteen minutes.
- While this is on the oven, you can prepare the sauce by mixing the cranberries and other ingredients in a small sauce pan.
- Cook the sauce mix over medium heat until it is thoroughly heated.

- You can then place the meatballs in a serving bowl and pour the sauce on it.
- You are to serve with toothpicks.

Nutrients			Renal and Renal Diabetic Exchanges
•	Calories	108	One meat
•	Carbohydrates	9	One low potassium fruit
•	Protein	5	
•	Fat	6	
•	Sodium	38	
•	Phosphorus	44	
•	Potassium	98	

Zippy delight

Ingredients:

- One package of cream cheese 8 oz (softened)
- Half cup of margarine (softened)
- Three tablespoons of green onion (chopped)
- Two tablespoons of mayonnaise
- One tablespoon of vinegar
- One and half teaspoons of lemon juice
- One and half teaspoons of hot dry mustard

- One teaspoon of "horseradish"
- One teaspoon paprika
- Half teaspoon of garlic powder
- Half teaspoon of tarragon
- A sprinkle of cayenne pepper

Serving mode: Two tablespoons per serving

Directions:

Blend all ingredients until they are thoroughly mix. You can serve with unsalted crackers or better still raw vegetables.

Nutrients		Renal and Renal Diabetic Exchanges
• Calories	155	One Low Potassium
• Carbohydrates	2	
• Protein	2	Vegetable
• Fat	16	Three Fat
• Sodium	133	
• Phosphorus	28	
• Potassium	43	

Breakfasts

Ingredients:

- Biscuits one and the half cups flour
- Two teaspoons of baking powder
- Two tablespoons of margarine
- 1/3 cup of liquid of non-dairy creamer
- 1/3 cup of water

Gravy

- 6 oz of ground beef
- Half teaspoon of sage
- Half teaspoon of pepper
- Half teaspoon basil
- Half teaspoon of garlic powder
- Two tablespoons of margarine
- Two tablespoons of cornstarch
- One cup of liquid of non-dairy creamer

Serving mode: Two Biscuits and 1/3 Cup Gravy Per Serving

Directions:

- The biscuits processing involves, mixing flour and baking powder in a bowl.
- Add margarine until mixture looks like a coarse meal.
- Then you can add creamer and water, you will mix it to form dough.
- Place on a floured surface for about 10 times.
- Roll dough out and cut into 8 biscuits.

- You are to bake on a well-greased baking sheet at 450°F for about 10 to 12 minutes until it turns golden.
- To make gravy, you can mix grounded beef with spices in a bowl.
- Put the Brown beef in a skillet and heat over medium heat. Drain. place aside.
- Right in the same skillet, you would melt margarine over a minimal heat.
- Get a small bowl, mix it with cornstarch and add1/4 cup creamer until it becomes smooth.
- You can then add the remaining creamer and stir the mixture until it becomes smooth.
- You then add the mixture to margarine in skillet and cook over a minimal heat and keep stirring constantly, until the mixture thickens and starts to bubbles.
- Add the beef and heat it thoroughly.
- You can serve it with biscuits.

Nutrients			Renal and Renal Diabetic Exchanges
•	Calories	524	One Meat
•	Carbohydrates	51	Two Starch
•	Protein	13	One non-dairy milk
•	Fat	31	
•	Sodium	525	
•	Phosphorus	311	Substitute
•	Potassium	393	Four fat

French toast delight

Ingredients:

- Three eggs
- 3/4 of cup milk
- One tablespoon of sugar
- One teaspoon of vanilla
- Half teaspoon cinnamon (optional)
- Six slices of French bread, you are to cut diagonally to about 1 inch thick
- One tablespoon of margarine

Serving mode: Two Slices per Serving

Directions:

- Beat the eggs, and then add milk, sugar, vanilla and cinnamon "optional" mix them together in large bowl, stir well until sugar dissolves.
- You can soak bread in egg mixture until it becomes saturated.
- You can then Heat the margarine in skillet until it's melted. You can then cook the bread over medium heat until it turns golden brown; you are to leave it for about 12 minutes on each side of the bread.
- You are to serve it with sprinkled powdered sugar and with pan-cake (optional).

Nutrient   Renal   and
                                                      Renal Diabetic

		Exchanges
• Calories	365	Two Starch
• Carbohydrates	47	One Meat
• Protein	15	One Milk
• Fat	13	
• Sodium	551	Half high
• Phosphorus	222	Calorie
• Potassium	206	One salt

Fruit and Oat Pancakes Delight

Ingredients:

• Half cup of rolled oats

• One cup of flour

• One to Eight-oz of can fruit cocktail (undrained)

• Half cup of liquid (non-dairy) creamer

• Half teaspoon of baking powder

• One egg or better still 1/4 cup liquid of egg as a substitute

• One tablespoon of margarine

Serving mode: Serve two Pancakes per serving

Directions:

• Mix all the ingredients except margarine in a bowl.

• You are to melt the margarine in a wide skillet.

• You can then drop the batter into skillet (1/4 cup per pancake) and then cook on a medium heat until the pancakes are well cooked and dry around the edges.

• Flip the pancakes with a spatula and then fry until the pancakes becomes golden brown at the bottom.

Nutrient			Renal and Renal Diabetic Exchanges
• Calories	262		Two Starch
• Carbohydrates	41		One Medium Potassium
• Protein	7		
• Fat	8		Fruit
• Sodium	152		
• Phosphorus	198		One Fat
• Potassium	186		

Mexican mix (brunch eggs)

Ingredients:

• Two tablespoons of margarine
• Half cup of nicely chopped onion
• Two of cloves garlic (crushed)
• One and half cups of frozen corn (defroze)
• One and half teaspoons of ground cumin
• 1/8 teaspoon of cayenne pepper
• Eight eggs, all beaten, or rather two cups of low-cholesterol egg as a substitute
• Two cups of unsalted corn chips

• Two tablespoons of well chopped pimiento
Serving mode: You are to serve only half cup per serving
Directions:
• In a large cooking pot, fry ⬚uickly in hot oil the onion and garlic in margarine until the gets onion soft.
• You can then add corn, cumin and cayenne.
• Then you stir to mix properly.
• You can then pour in the eggs into the mix and cook it over minimal heat, you can then stir occasionally, until the eggs are properly fried and set.
• You are to arrange corn chips on a wide platter.
• Pour the egg mixture on chips and sprinkle it with pimiento. Serve fresh hot immediately.

Nutrients			Renal and Renal Diabetic Exchanges
•	Calories	214	One Meat
•	Carbohydrates	13	One Starch
•	Protein	9	One Medium Potassium
•	Fat	14	
•	Sodium	147	
•	Phosphorus	91	Vegetable
•	Potassium	240	One Fat

Triple pepper quiche

Ingredients:

- One tablespoon of margarine
- One fresh green pepper (You are to cut it in strips)
- One sweet red pepper (You are to cut it in strips)
- One sweet yellow pepper (You are to cut it in strips)
- Four eggs or rather use one cup of low cholesterol egg
- Half cup of liquid (non-dairy) creamer
- Half cup of water
- Half teaspoon of basil
- 1/8 teaspoon of cayenne pepper
- One to Nine inch of pie shell (unbaked)

Serving mode: 1/8 of Quiche per serving

Directions:

- In a large cooking pot, you are to sauté the pepper strips in margarine until it gets soft but make sure it's not limp.
- Mix eggs or egg substitute, creamer, water, basil and cayenne in a bowl.
- With your spoon pour peppers into unbaked pie shell.
- Now pour the egg mixture over the peppers.
- Then bake at a temperature of 375°F for about 50 to 55 minutes until you the knife inserted in the center comes out unsoiled or rather clean.
- Let the delicacy stay for about ten minutes before you can serve.

Nutrients   Renal

Exchanges

- Calories 201
- Carbohydrates 14
- Protein 5
- Fat 14
- Sodium 222
- Phosphorus 50
- Potassium 163

One Starch

One Low Potassium vegetable

Two Fat

Renal Diabetic Exchanges:

One Starch

One medium potassium vegetable

Two Fat

Soups And Salads

Bow-tie pasta salad

Ingredients:

- Two cups of cooked bowtie like pasta
- 1/4 cup of chopped celery
- Two tablespoons of chopped green pepper
- Two tablespoons of shredded carrots
- Two tablespoons of minced onion
- 1/8 teaspoon of pepper
- 2/3 cup of mayonnaise
- Half teaspoon of sugar
- One tablespoon of lemon juice

Serving mode: Just 1/3 Cup per serving
Directions:
- You are to mix the pasta celery, green pepper carrot and onion inside a bowl
- In another small bowl blend the pepper, mayonnaise, sugar and lemon juice together until it becomes smooth.
- Now pour the pasta over and vegetables and mix them very well until they are well coated.
- And then chill in the fridge.

Nutrients   Renal   and
                                    Renal Diabetic

- Calories   189
- Carbohydrates   12
- Protein   2
- Fat   15
- Sodium   111
- Phosphorus   31
- Potassium   61

Con Carne with Chili

Ingredients:

• One lb of lean grounded beef
• One cup of chopped onion
• Half cup of chopped green pepper
• Six oz of unsalted tomato paste
• Two tablespoons of chili powder
• One teaspoon of garlic powder
• Half teaspoon of grounded cumin
• Half teaspoon of paprika
• One ⬚uart water

Serving mode: Re⬚uires only one cup per serving
Directions:
• Get a large pot and brown the ground beef inside.
• Make sure you drain the fat.
• And then add onion and green pepper.
• You are to cook the onion until it is transparent.
• And then add the remaining ingredients and simmer for one and half hours.

- What to do before serving it, try to measure chili and add more water to make Five cups.
- Then heat through till it's ready.

Nutrients		Renal and Renal Diabetic Exchanges
• Calories	254	
• Carbohydrates	11	Three Meat
• Protein	21	
• Fat	14	Two Medium Potassium vegetable
• Sodium	118	
• Phosphorus	182	
• Potassium	638	

Cheese salad (cottage)

Ingredients:

- Two lb creamed cheese (cottage)
- One to Six-oz of canned crushed pineapple juice (drained)
- One to Eight-oz of carton whipped cream
- One to Three-oz of package (Jell O) you can choose the lime or raspberry flavor, depending on your preference

Serving mode: Half cup per serving is required
Directions:
- Pour the dry (Jell O ®) into the cottage cheese.
- And then add the drained pineapple.
- Carefully fold in whipped cream.
- And finally refrigerate.

Nutrients			Renal and Renal Diabetic Exchanges
• Calories	191		
• Carbohydrates	5		Two Meat
• Protein	17		Half Low Potassium
• Fat	11		
• Sodium	348		
• Phosphorus	105		Fruit
• Potassium	122		One Salt

Frozen salad (cranberry)

Ingredients:

- One to Eight-oz packaged creamed cheese
- Half pint of whipping cream (whipped)
- Half teaspoon of vanilla extract
- One to Sixteen-oz of can cranberry sauce
Serving mode: 3 x 3 - inch piece per serving
Directions:

• You are to whip the cream cheese with a beater until it gets fluffy.

• Carefully fold in vanilla and the whipped cream and then the cranberry sauce.

• After that you put it into a 9 x 9 - inch container.

• Freeze it

• You are to cut it into s◻uares and serve frozen.

Nutrients		Renal and Renal Diabetic Exchanges
• Calories	255	
• Carbohydrates	21	Half Starch
• Protein	2.5	One Low Potassium Fruit
• Fat	19	
• Sodium	99	
• Phosphorus	46	Three Fat
• Potassium	63	

Cranberry salad

Ingredients:

• Two to Three-oz of package raspberry

• One can of whole cranberry sauce (please note not jellied)

• One cup of apples, it should be peeled and chopped

• One cup of celery, it should be chopped

• Half cup of unsalted nuts

Serving mode: Half cup per serving

Directions:

- You will mix package raspberry according to directions in the pack.
- When the mixture is cool and looks like syrup, you can add the cranberry sauce, apples, celery and nuts.
- After you done with all that you can then refrigerate until firm.

Nutrients and nutritional facts (According to the chosen packages in your raspberry)		Renal and Renal Diabetic Exchanges
- Calories	179	
- Carbohydrates	34	One Low Potassium Fruit
- Protein	2.4	
- Fat	5	
- Sodium	75	One Starch
- Phosphorus	93	
- Potassium	26	One Fat

Corn soup cream

Ingredients:

- Two tablespoons of margarine
- Two tablespoons of flour
- 1/8 teaspoon of pepper
- One cup of water
- One cup of liquid non-dairy creamer
- Two of jars (Jar measurement: 128 g each) of strained (cream-style) corn baby food

111

Serving mode: One cup per serving
Directions:
• Place the saucepan on a minimal heat, and then melt the margarine.
• Then you add flour and pepper
• Stir it well until it becomes smooth
• Gradually add water and non-dairy creamer
• Cook the mixture until it start to bubble
• Stir while you add in corn

Nutrients			Renal and Renal Diabetic Exchanges
• Calories	245		Two Low Potassium
• Carbohydrates	22		
• Protein	3		Vegetable
• Fat	16		One Non-dairy Milk
• Sodium	164		
• Phosphorus	85		Substitute
• Potassium	238		One Fat

Crab Soup with cream

Ingredients:

• One tablespoon of unsalted margarine
• Chopped half bulb Onion (medium)
• Half lb imitation crabmeat (shredded)
• One quart low sodium chicken broth

- One cup of non-dairy coffee creamer
- Two tablespoons of cornstarch
- 1/8 teaspoon of dill weed

Serving mode: One cup of per serving

Directions:

- On a moderate heat you are to melt margarine in a large cooking pot .
- And then add onion, cook and stir at the same time until gets soft.
- Add your crab meat and then cook for about three minutes continuously stir the mixture.
- Add your chicken broth and boil it.
- Remember to reduce the heat to minimal.
- Mix them in a bowl with non-dairy creamer and cornstarch. Continue stirring until it becomes smooth.
- And then add to soup and you can increase the heat to moderate, while you continue stirring, until the mixture becomes boiled and thickens.
- Stir and add dill weed.

Nutrients			Renal and Renal Diabetic Exchanges
•	Calories	87	
•	Carbohydrates	7	One Low Potassium
•	Protein	4	
•	Fat	5	Vegetable
•	Sodium	241	One Fat
•	Phosphorus	82	

- Potassium   80

Chicken Salad with Lemon Curry

Ingredients:

- 1/4 cup oil
- Four tablespoons of frozen lemonade concentrate (thawed)
- 1/4 teaspoon of ground ginger
- 1/4 teaspoon of curry powder
- 1/8 teaspoon of garlic powder
- One and half cups of cooked diced chicken
- One and half cups of grapes
- Half cup of sliced celery

Serving mode: One cup per serving

Directions:

- Get a large bowl; add oil, lemonade concentrate and spices.
- Add the remaining ingredients and slightly toss around.

And then chill

Nutrients			Renal and Renal Diabetic Exchanges
• Calories	307		Two Meat
• Carbohydrates	15		One Starch
• Protein	17		Two Fat
• Fat	20		

- Sodium   57
- Phosphorus   119
- Potassium   235

Salad Niçoise with Pasta

Ingredients:

• Four cups of cooked small shell macaroni
• One tablespoon of olive oil
• Two cups of fresh green beans, you are to cut into 1-inch pieces
• Half cup of lemon juice
• 1/3 cup of olive oil
• Two teaspoons of dry mustard
• One tablespoon of chopped fresh parsley
• One teaspoon of basil
• One 7-3/4-oz of can tuna that is packed in water (drained)
• Five green onions, that is chopped, with added tops
• 1/4 teaspoon of pepper

Serving mode: One and half cups per serving
Directions:
• You are to toss pasta with one tablespoon of olive oil all in a bowl.
• After that, you set it aside.
• Put Blanch green beans into boiling water and boil for two minutes.

- After then you transfer it to a colander and chill running water and then drain.
- Get a large bowl, and mix beans, lemon juice, 1/3 cup of olive oil, mustard, parsley and basil together.
- Add tuna, green onions, pasta and pepper.
- Toss the mixture, and then cover it, allow to it chill for at least One to Two hours

Nutrients		Renal and Renal Diabetic Exchanges
Calories	304	
Carbohydrates	25	Two Meat
Protein	15	One Starch
Fat	16	
Sodium	135	One Low Potassium
Phosphorus	293	
Potassium	293	Vegetable
		One Fat

Seed dressing poppy style

Ingredients:

- 1/4 cup of and two tablespoons of wine vinegar
- Two tablespoons of lemon juice
- Five tablespoons of sugar

- One teaspoon of dry mustard

- 1/4 small onion (minced)

- Half cup of oil

- And one tablespoon of poppy seed

Serving mode: It is 2/3 Cup per serving

Directions:

Combine all the ingredients together. Serve this delicacy with salad of your choice.

Nutrients			Renal and Renal Diabetic Exchanges
•	Calories	82	
•	Carbohydrates	5	Two Fat
•	Protein	0	
•	Fat	7	
•	Sodium	0	
•	Phosphorus	8	
•	Potassium	18	

Meat, Chicken And Sea Food

Halibut baked

Ingredients:

- One and half lb of halibut steaks
- 1/4 cup of mayonnaise
- 3/4 cup of bread crumbs
- Lemon slices soaked in paprika

Serving mode: Three ounces per serving

Directions:

- You are to preheat in an oven with a heat of 400°F.
- Then remove the steaks out of the bone in center, and cut into serving size pieces.
- The next thing to do is to rub and cover it with mayonnaise. Then deep in bread crumbs.
- You are getting the steaks ready for making now, so place in a baking pan rubbed with butter.
- You are to bake in preheated oven of about fifteen minutes Then carefully place them on heated serving platter.
- And then finally garnish with lemon slices.

Nutrients		Renal and Renal Diabetic Exchanges
• Calories	205	
• Carbohydrates	8	Three Meat
• Protein	22	One Milk
• Fat	9	
• Sodium	176	

- Phosphorus   233
- Potassium   456

Shrimp with Broiled Garlic

Ingredients:

• One lb of shrimp still in its shells
• Half cup of an unsalted margarine (melt the margarine)
• Two teaspoons of lemon juice
• Two tablespoons of chopped onion
• One clove of garlic (minced)
• 1/8 teaspoon of pepper
• One tablespoon of fresh parsley (chop the pepper)
Serving mode: You are to serve about two and half Ounces of Shrimp per Serving
Directions:
• You are to preheat broiler.
• And then wash, peel and dry the shrimp.
• Get a shallow baking pan and pour the margarine in and then add the various ingredients like lemon juice, onion, garlic and pepper.
• You are to add shrimp and toss very well to coat.
• Broil for five minutes.
• And then turn and broil for another five more minutes. Then finally serve the delicacy on platter with strained pan juices.
• And then finally sprinkle your parsley to garnish.

Nutrients   Renal   and

- Calories   264
- Carbohydrates 2
- Protein   19
- Fat   20
- Sodium   135
- Phosphorus   192
- Potassium   189

Pork chops (cajun)

Ingredients:

- 1/4 teaspoon of paprika
- 1/4 teaspoon of garlic powder
- 1/4 teaspoon of thyme
- 1/4 teaspoon of dry mustard
- 1/4 teaspoon of ground sage
- 1/4 teaspoon of ground cumin
- 1/8 teaspoon of pepper
- Four pork chops that is cut into half-inch thick (Four oz each)
- One small onion that is sliced
- One tablespoon of margarine
- One teaspoon of parsley flakes

• 1/8 teaspoon of garlic powder
• Two to Three drops hot pepper sauce
Serving mode: One chop per serving

Directions:
• Mix paprika, 1/4 teaspoon of garlic powder, mustard, thyme, sage, cumin and then pepper on clean waxed paper.
• And the coat very well both sides of the pork chops with this mixture.
• Arrange the coated pork chops in one layer placed on an eight-inch square microwave safe dish.
• Sprinkle pork chop with onion slices.
• And then cover with waxed paper.
• You are to Microwave on high for about five minutes.
• And then place on Rotate dish and microwave on low heat (30% should be ok) for about twenty five to thirty minutes or rather until the delicacy gets tender, make sure you rotate once during this period.
• Keep the pork chop aside while you prepare the sauce.
• Mix the margarine, parsley, 1/8 teaspoon of garlic powder and pepper sauce all in a small glass bowl.
• Set the Microwave on high for about 30 to 40 seconds until the mixture is melted.
• Pour the sauce over chops before serving.

Nutrients			Renal and Renal Diabetic Exchanges
•	Calories	234	Three Meat
•	Carbohydrates	3	One Medium Potassium
•	Protein	22	
•	Fat	16	Vegetable
•	Sodium	75	One Fat
•	Phosphorus	245	
•	Potassium	447	

Do not go yet; One last thing to do

If you enjoyed this book or found it useful I'd be very grateful if you'd post a short review on it. Your support really does make a difference and I read all the reviews personally so I can get your feedback and make this book even better.

Thanks again for your support!

Part 2

Introduction To The Renal Diet!

A renal diet is an eating plan conceived to help people who suffer from renal diseases. It can expand the effectiveness of treatment by lowering the level of waste products in their blood.

This diet is designed to avoid stressing kidneys, and it provides useful nutrients and energy to the body.

The diet is based on some basic rules.

The main rule is that it must be a healthy and balanced diet, rich in fibers, natural grains, carbohydrates, omega 3 fats, vitamins and fluids. Protein should be present but not excessively, they are essential to rebuild tissues but cannot be exceeding in this diet as excessive quantities of proteins should be broken down by the body into carbohydrates and nitrates. Moreover, as nitrates are not used by the body, they should be excreted through the kidneys.

Salts are kept to a minimum and electrolyte levels of blood are checked on a regular basis and are then balanced accordingly. Please inform your doctor before starting the diet.

Carbohydrates are important for energy and need to be taken in the right quantities. However, you should avoid refined ones. You should try to use as many whole grains and unrefined forms of carbohydrates as possible.

Table salt should be used only for cooking and remember that excessive salt causes retention and stress to the kidneys. Salty foods should be avoided as well: no sausages, no snacks, no tinned food.

There is also the level of phosphorus which needs to be monitored carefully, avoiding colored drinks like colas and food with a high level of potassium such as bananas, citrus fruits, apricots, dark leafy green vegetables should be avoided too, especially if blood levels rise.

Take into consideration also Omega 3 fats which are important in your diet but avoid trans-fats and hydrolyzed fats.

The proper renal diet can really help kidneys functioning longer, and it has only more restrictions on proteins and table salt, while restrictions to phosphorous and potassium can be needed if the levels of blood rise and the signs of accumulation become too evident.

Hereafter we are going to have a look at the benefits and dangers in many foods and nutrients.

Food And Nutrients In The Renal Diet

Protein: the best you can do is to talk to your doctor when it comes to dealing with proteins in your diet, as their presence could vary according to physical activity levels and, in any case, you should limit your protein intake if your kidneys are damaged. We still need some protein so we need to chose which are the best: cut dairy and red meat, as they are often too high in fats and sodium.

Chicken is better than red meat, but organic chicken is preferable in general. Fish is a fundamental source of proteins, and it is strong in anti-inflammatory action, which is beneficial to your kidneys.

Also soy and tofu are recommended: when taken on a regular basis, they even show a slow progression of kidney damage.

There are also three minerals which need to be avoided in your diet as kidneys need to filter the blood of these minerals to achieve the correct levels, but when kidneys are damaged this does not happen correctly, so the levels can higher and become too dangerous: potassium, phosphorus, and sodium. We will try to understand how each of these minerals can be dangerous and how to avoid them.

More in general, all diets should avoid excessive levels of sodium, as it increases blood pressure, which is a direct cause of kidneys diseases as it forces the kidneys to filter more, increasing their stress. And more kidney pressure causes high blood pressure, so this is like a dangerous circle.

Do not salt your food too much, avoid fast foods and takeaways, as they use salt a lot to increase flavor, but this is dangerous for your health. There are also foods containing hidden quantities of sodium such as processed meats, frozen and canned food, sports drinks, and snacks.

Potassium then is very important for us as it is required for nerve, cardiac functions, and fluid balance, but when its level is not the right one in our body, this may be a danger for kidneys functions. Potassium level builds up in the blood level and may end up with cardiovascular problems. We consequently need to reduce potassium in the renal diet, and we can verify this by blood sampling. We will need then to reduce the use of tomatoes, potatoes, bananas, nuts, seeds, chocolate, pumpkin, and avoid some vegetables or remove it from plants.

Phosphorus is another vital mineral for bones and teeth as it is key to the regulation of calcium, but for people suffering from kidneys damages the excessive presence of it in the blood can lead to osteoporosis and high blood pressure.

Basically, the renal diet is like an alkaline diet, as there is a need to balance pH in the blood, which is not well balanced when there is kidney disease. There is a need to avoid acidic foods from the diet. It is also true that acidity contributes to many health issues such as kidney stones, urinary problems, high blood pressure, and reduced immunity levels.

Sometimes, however, with the alkaline diet, it is not so easy to determine which foods are really acidic: let's take the lemon, for example. It tastes acidic, but it produces a real alkaline effect once it is digested.

It is right to think that most foods that are considered unhealthy are also acidic (meat, sugary treats, alcohol, wheat, most dairy products), but some acidic foods are right in the renal diet (for example olive oil, fish, soymilk, and nuts).

Following the alkaline diet, you need to consume 80% of alkaline products and 20% of acidic foods. You can, of course, test your urinary health and pH every day and then change this balance with a 60% alkaline and 40% acid.

Most alkaline foods are considered suitable for the renal diet, and they are fruits, vegetables, brown rice, green juices, tofu, sprouts, herbal teas.

The essential renal diet is crucial to your kidneys' health and to protect them from any possible future damage, and you can also add herbs and nutrients which can improve kidneys' health.

A Diet For Patients With Renal Problems

This diet is highly recommended for patients with renal problems, and what we know is that only 25% of nephrons are needed to maintain healthy renal functions. That is, it takes a long time before a kidney disease may appear, but it is also true that when we have symptoms, it means that true kidney damage is already happening.

Nitrogenous waste products, impaired excretion of electrolytes, vitamin deficiencies, and continued catabolism are the main reasons for continuous diet adjustments. Wasting syndrome is the main problem. Clients with renal issues consistently lose weight; they low down muscle mass and lose adipose tissues.

The goal in this type of nutrition is to maintain a balance of electrolytes, minerals, fluids. Dialysis on its own is not able to remove and filter the wastes in the body. The body needs to be helped in managing the accumulated waste.

The regulation of sodium, for example, is very important. When kidneys waste salt, sodium must be risen to replace it. When kidneys retain sodium, so the fluid status must be monitored to get the right info on sodium needs.

Patients and family members' quality of life are always badly affected by renal problems and therapies. All the therapies such as dialysis or also hemodialysis can affect the psychological aspects of life.

What you will find hereafter is not simply a diet but a careful analysis to approach the symptoms of renal disease and to maintain good energy levels for your daily activities. There is also information about the exact amount of proteins, electrolytes, minerals, and fluids allowed for the patients.

Guidelines For A Good Renal Diet

Hereafter you will find indications on the quantity of salt to be introduced in your blood to control these levels through the food you eat. Every patient is different, and this depends on the severity of the malfunctioning, on the fact that you might be overweight or on the electrolytes in your blood: all these factors must be taken into consideration to understand if you need dialysis or not. When there is renal failure, the levels of salt in our blood can become really critical, without balance the renal diet should help you restore this balance and put your kidneys less under stress.

Renal diet guidelines are based on blood test results and on a healthy balanced diet. It tries to limit the quantity of salt intake. Fluids also are restricted if your kidneys are unable to excrete sufficient water. Proteins as well are at the minimum in order for the urea wastes to be kept low.

The salts that need to be less used and be restricted are:

Sodium, which causes high blood tension and fluid retention. There is the need for "no added salt" recipes, so you should avoid processed food, sausages, sauce, ketchup, and many canned foods.

Phosphorus cannot be removed by dialysis so it can be a big problem. Its levels must be constantly kept under control by diet and medication. So you should avoid dairy products, beans, peas, beer and cola drinks.

Potassium needs to be restricted if its level in the blood is high. So you should avoid apricots, orange juice, bananas, avocados, beets, spinach, and others.

Proteins should only be taken in small quantities. You should avoid meat, fish, eggs, and dairy products.

Fluids can be restricted if there is water retention. You should thus avoid too high quantities of beverages, soups, water, and juices.

Carbohydrates are energy food and should not be eliminated unless you are diabetic or overweight. You should also take vitamins and antioxidant supplements to help the immune system.

The renal diet is meant to decrease the workload on damaged kidneys and to maintain their health and function. It is imperative in this case to consult your doctor.

Renal Disease And The Diet

Consult your doctor as often as you can: the kidneys are your body toxin's filter, and you should always try to clean your blood from toxins and preservatives in food.

Try not to eat irresponsibly (foods, drinks and even the air you breath) as many elements can be turned into something bad like formaldehyde due to a chemical reaction and morphing phase, which can lead to renal failure, cancer or various other problems.

Renal failure happens when your kidneys are not able to get rid of toxins and wastes in your blood, and this is called chronic kidney disease" or "chronic renal failure."

This is a progressive problem, and it can be found out, treated, the diet changed, and it might also be possible to resolve what is the cause of the problem. It usually takes a long time to get to renal failure and you certainly to want to reach it because this would require dialysis treatments to save your life, to clean the blood and remove the toxins in the blood using a machine because your body can no longer do this job. Without treatments, you could die a very painful death. It can be the result of long periods of high blood pressure, irresponsible diet, diabetes.

The renal diet uses a low quantity of proteins and phosphorus, sodium, and this will control the toxins in your blood, helping your kidneys functions. If you adjust your diet very fast and early, you could prevent total renal failure.

The Renal Diet For Diabetic Patients

For diabetics who suffer from renal disease, there is a specific diet known as diabetic renal diet. Very often, this diet is also conceived for diabetics who want to avoid incurring in renal diseases.

Diabetics and patients with renal disease often have problems in eating the right food.

The aim of this diet is to have glucose levels within the right range. This is possible by not missing any meals, by having a regular diet, by eating low glycemic carbohydrates, in order to help the body always have the same level of glucose and low glycemic foods are grains bread, sweet potatoes, and brown rice. However, if the diet is for renal problems, you should also avoid sweet potatoes and grain bread, as they are rich in potassium.

People with renal problems, as we have already seen, should avoid food rich in potassium phosphorus and sodium. Since sodium is often present, patients should look carefully at labels, and dietitians should advise patients to avoid sodas with dark colors, coffee, and drinks with too much sodium for diabetics with renal problems.

Unsweetened teas, water, and clear diet sodas are allowed. As for vegetables, broccoli, cauliflowers, beets, eggplant, and cabbage are recommended for their vitamin-rich features, together with their low potassium and carbohydrates content. You should then avoid meat such as sausage, bacon, and organ meats.

Also, avoid canned vegetables as they are rich in sodium: nutritionists will also guide you on portion sizes to help your blood glucose control.

Many people suffering from renal problems also have diabetes. The main goal for diabetic diets is to maintain the right level of glucose in your blood. This can be done by:

- Eating carbohydrates with a low glycemic index (GI) such as grains, unrefined foods, most fruits and vegetables, legumes, sweet potatoes (only in some quantities), nuts.

- White bread, sugar, confectionaries, drinks with added sugar should be avoided

- Eating small frequent meals is a good habit. Don't go long periods without eating and don't do huge meals or even worse, do not skip meals.

The renal diet then tries not to stress kidneys, and this can be done by:

- Limiting daily intake of proteins: an excess of proteins need to be broken into carbohydrates and nitrites which, in the form of urea, can be destroyed by urine as it causes stress on already damaged kidneys.

- Limiting table salt and do not use a salt replacement as they contain potassium.

- Reduce also potassium and phosphates, including apricots, avocado, bananas, kiwi, watermelon, peaches, prunes as phosphorus avoid legumes, dairy products, dried legumes, shellfish, organ meats.

The renal diet for diabetics food pyramid:

This is a pyramid (divided into 5 groups) which indicates appropriate eating, where the larger group is made up of grains, rice, beans, starchy vegetables.

Then we have a smaller group including fruits and vegetables

A smaller quantity is dedicated to food with less fat and salt. If you drink alcohol, take it in moderate quantities. Choose food high in fibers and vitamins and minerals, such as whole grain and be physically active at least 30 minutes a day.

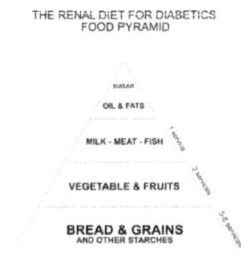

THE RENAL DIET FOR DIABETICS
FOOD PYRAMID

SUGAR

OIL & FATS

MILK - MEAT - FISH

VEGETABLE & FRUITS

BREAD & GRAINS
AND OTHER STARCHES

Eat frequently with small and repeated meals, when you wake up in the morning eat your first meal and then every 2-3 hours, taking your last meal at bedtime.

PLEASE NOTE:

If you plan your full week it will be easier for you to follow the diet, always fill up the plate with half of it with vegetables and salads, then the other half with proteins or carbohydrates.

No salt, and instead of it use fresh herbs, spices, onions, garlic, lemon juice.

For smaller meals eat whole grain cereals, crackers or bread, fruit, a glass of skim milk, nuts, yogurt, plenty of salads, or a small quantity of cottage cheese.

This diet can be powerful in both controlling renal failure and diabetes. Stick to your diet, and you will feel better and healthier.

How To Manage Diabetes And Renal Diseases Effectively

Diabetic renal diet is a subject of interest as diabetes mellitus is one of the most common extrarenal diseases affecting the kidneys.

Diabetes mellitus leads to diabetic nephropathy in 30% of cases and to its end stage.

Researchers estimate that 25-30% of diabetes mellitus patients end up with end-stage renal diseases 10 to 20 years beginning insulin therapy.

Renal disease can also happen to non-insulin dependent diabetic patients. The incidence of protein in urine presence is about 25% after 20 years of diabetes.

The diabetic renal diet is conceived to help metabolic control in these types of patients. By controlling diabetes mellitus, we can also control the worsening situation of kidneys and prevent end-stage renal disease.

The kidney metabolizes 30-40% of insulin, and as the renal functions decline, the degradation of insulin also decreases, leading to a lower insulin need. Renal failure can be identified when the patient is evaluated for recurrent insulin reactions.

Renal disease can be controlled by

- checking hypertension carefully

- adjusting insulin therapy

- restricting protein in your diet.

However, renal failure appears within 5 to 10 years after the first appear of proteinuria (protein in urine).

The following are some recommendations for patients with diabetes mellitus.

- total calories: to maintain reasonable weight in adults, meet increased needs in children, adolescents, pregnant and lactating women and people recovering from catabolic illness

- caloric distribution: 50 to 70 % of carbohydrates, 20 to 30% of proteins, 20 to 30% of fats

- cholesterol limited under 300mg/day or less

- sodium below 300mg/day less for people with hypertension and renal complications

- alcohol: a very moderate amount

- vitamin and mineral supplements: to be given to individuals with low caloric diets (1200 kcal/day)

The diet for an individual with diabetes can only be a dietary prescription based on nutrition assessment and treatment goals. The diabetic renal diet can be a good guideline to control and manage diabetes mellitus, which may then go into renal diseases.

Renal Diet – The Meals

The following diet is divided by:

Breakfast

Lunch

Dinner

Desserts

Extra and minimal meals for different moments of the day.

You will have a list of ingredients, a paragraph dedicated to "how to prepare" the recipe and a list of nutrients per portion.

All recipes, divided by the different moments of the day, are listed in alphabetic order.

Breakfast

Avocado Toast With Eggs

Ingredients
2 slices of whole-grain bread
1 tablespoon of parsley
½ Hass avocado
1 tablespoon of lime juice
1/8 teaspoon salt
2 eggs
2 tablespoons of crumbled feta cheese
1/8 teaspoon of ground black pepper

How to prepare the recipe

Toast the bread slices and cut the parsley into thin cubes or slices, setting it apart.
Mash half of avocado with a fork after you have

removed the skin and add lime juice and a bit of salt. Spread this mixture on the toast slices.

Prepare a dish to be put in the oven at medium heat by spreading it with non-stick cooking spray. Break the eggs in the dish and cook them until you are satisfied with their consistency. Put the eggs onto the top of the avocado on the toast and put some feta cheese on the eggs, add the chopped parsley and the ground black pepper.

Nutrients per portion

225 calories
12 g protein
15 g carbohydrates
13 g fat
195 mg cholesterol
404 mg sodium
311 mg potassium
209 mg phosphorus
107 mg calcium
4.3 fiber

Asparagus And Cheese Crepes With Parsley

Ingredients

12 asparagus
4 ounces of soft cheese
1/2 teaspoon of black pepper
1/3 cup of flour
½ glass of water

¼ bowl of cream
1 egg
2 egg whites
4 tablespoons of butter
1 piece of parsley
1 teaspoon of lemon juice

How to prepare the recipe

Cook the asparagus for 6 to 8 minutes
Mix the softened cream cheese with the parsley, spices
and lemon juice to prepare a sauce.
Put then together flour with water, egg, egg whites,
and 2 tablespoons of butter already melted: mix
everything to prepare a batter.
Prepare 8 to 10-inch crepe by melting the butter taken
from 1/2 tablespoon, adding 1/3 of cup crepe batter
and turn the pan to spread the batter. Cook it on both
sides, cool it and repeat in order to prepare 4 crepes.
Insert the cheese in the crepes that you are willing to
roll afterward, putting inside also the asparagus.
Put them in the fridge for 1 hour, and after cut the
crepes rolls into 3-4 pieces before putting them on the
table.

Nutrients per portion

305 calories
10 g protein
16 g carbohydrates
24 g fat
114 mg cholesterol
245 mg sodium
355 mg potassium
140 mg phosphorus
95 mg calcium
2.8 fiber

Baked French Toast In Batter

Ingredients

4 slices Italian bread
4 cups of non-enriched rice milk
2 cups liquid low cholesterol egg substitute
½ cup sugar
4 spoons unsalted margarine (tablespoons)
1 teaspoon almond extract
1 teaspoon cinnamon
Non-calories sweetener

How to prepare the recipe

Spread margarine or non-stick cooking spray in the pan
on the bottom and sides of it.
Put sliced bread on the bottom of the pan
Beat non-enriched rice milk, egg substitute, melted

margarine, sugar, almond extract, and cinnamon all together in a cup and pour over bread slices.

Cover everything with plastic wrap and put it in the fridge for one night.

Preheat oven at 350°F (around 170 é Celsius)

Bake for 50 minutes until the knife can cut easily and serve warm.

Sprinkle with non-calories sweetener if you wish.

Nutrients per portion

450 calories
16 g protein
65 g carbohydrates
14 g fat
0 mg cholesterol
390 mg sodium
220 mg potassium
110 mg phosphorus
86 mg calcium
0.8 fiber

Benedicts' Eggs Muffins

Ingredients

4 ounces of bacon in slices
3 glasses of water
2 muffins
1 tablespoon vinegar
1 tablespoon of lemon juice
4 eggs

1/2 cup of unsalted butter
3 egg yolks
pepper
paprika

How to prepare the recipe

Place the bacon in 2 cups of boiling water for 5 minutes
in order to demineralize it. Put it on a towel and dry it
to absorb the moisture. Cut the muffins and toast
them. Cut the bacon and place it on top of each muffin
slice. Put vinegar with water in a big bowl and boil it,
reducing the heat slowly.
Break the eggs and put them into the water to poach
them. Cover and wait for 3 to 5 minutes for the eggs to
be ready. Remove the eggs and put them on the bacon
and muffin, cover it and keep it warm.
At a light heat beat the yolks and melt some butter,
adding this to the eggs with paprika and pepper. Add
some lemon juice and pour all on top of the muffins.

Nutrients per portion

415 calories
15 g protein
15 g carbohydrates
35 g fat
440 mg cholesterol
345 mg sodium
170 mg potassium
214 mg phosphorus

105 mg calcium
1.0 fiber

Blueberry Smoothie

Ingredients

1 cup of frozen blueberries
2 tablespoons of whey protein powder
¼ of Greek yogurt, non-fat yogurt
1/3 cup unsweetened vanilla with almond milk
2 strawberries
5 raspberries
1 tablespoon of fiber cereals
2 teaspoons of shredded coconut

How to prepare the recipe

Put the blueberries in a blender for 1 minute, add yogurt, protein powder and milk, blend all together until it is soft and scoop the mixture into a bowl. Top everything with sliced strawberries, raspberries, fiber cereals and shredded coconut. Add honey if you like it or a sweetener.

Nutrients per portion

225 calories
15 g protein
28 g carbohydrates
5 g fat
3 mg cholesterol

118 mg sodium
370 mg potassium
175 mg phosphorus
240 mg calcium
7.8 fiber

Cereals And Rice Cakes Mix

Ingredients

1cup of corn cereals
1 cup rice cereals
1/2 cup Cocoa cereals
1/2 cup of mini rice cakes (plain or apple cinnamon)

How to prepare the recipe

In a medium container mix all ingredients together and prepare separate portions.
Serve dry or with milk substitute.
Ask your doctor for a list of approved cereals.

Nutrients per portion

145 calories
2 g protein
32 g carbohydrates
1 g fat
0 mg cholesterol
235 mg sodium
70 mg potassium
50 mg phosphorus

96 mg calcium
1.0 fiber

Easy Crepe

Ingredients

3 eggs
1-1/3 whole milk
¾ all-purpose white flour
3 tablespoon butter

How to prepare the recipe

Mix both eggs and milk in a blender.
Add flour slowly and blend for 1 minute
Pour crepe batter in a bowl and add melted butter.
Heat a 8 inches crepe pan and coat pan with butter or
non-stick cooking spray all at medium heat.
Pour batter into the pan and make sure it lies evenly
moving the pan if necessary. The crepe will bubble.
Remove from pan when the crepe is golden, and its
edges are a bit brown.

Nutrients per portion

60 calories
3 g protein
6 g carbohydrates
3 g fat

46 mg cholesterol
29 mg sodium
50 mg potassium
45 mg phosphorus
31 mg calcium
0.1 fiber

Egg Cups

Ingredients

6 slices low sodium bacon
1/3 cup onion
1/3 cup mushrooms
1/3 cup bell pepper
12 large eggs
¼ teaspoon black pepper

How to prepare the recipe

Preheat the oven at 350°F. Line muffin tin with paper muffin wrappers. Bake bacon until it crisps. In a big bowl, crumble cooked bacon and mix it with dices of vegetables. Put the mixture into different cups, filling them by 2/3, leaving room to add the mixture itself.
In another recipient beat together both eggs and black pepper.
Pour egg mixture into each muffin cup. Leave ¼ inch at the top.

Bake 25 minutes until muffin has risen and are firm. Remove them from the pan and serve.

Nutrients per portion

80 calories
7 g protein
1 g carbohydrates
5 g fat
210 mg cholesterol
80 mg sodium
90 mg potassium
100 mg phosphorus
28 mg calcium
0.1 fiber

French Toast With Cinnamon Apple

Ingredients

1 pound loaf cinnamon
8 ounces crème cheese
1 or 2 apples
6 tablespoon unsalted butter
1 teaspoon ground cinnamon
8 eggs
1 e ¼ cup half and half creamer
1 e ¼ cup almond milk, unsweetened
¼ cup pancake syrup

How to prepare the recipe

Divide both bread and cream cheese into dices.
Remove peel and cut the apples into small cubes. Melt the butter.
Coat a 9" x 13" baking dish with cooking spray. Place half of the sliced bread into the dish and sprinkle the cream cheese dices over the bread, topping it with apple cubes. Spread the cinnamon on top with the rest of the bread.
In a pie dish beat the eggs with the half and half creamer, the milk, melted butter, and pancake syrup. Pour the mixture over the bread.
Cover your cooking dish with plastic wrap and press so that all the pieces are soaked. Refrigerate for 2 hours at least.
Preheat the oven at 325° F. Bake for 50 minutes and let it stand afterward for at least 10 minutes before serving. You can cut it into squares for up to 12 portions.
Put the pancake syrup on and add jam or cinnamon/raspberry applesauce if you like it.

Nutrients per portion

320 calories
9 g protein
27 carbohydrates
20 g fat
170 mg cholesterol
280 mg sodium

224 mg potassium
150 mg phosphorus
116 mg calcium
1.8 fiber

Grapefruit In Broiled Honey

Ingredients

1 grapefruit
2 teaspoons of honey
¼ teaspoon cinnamon

How to prepare the recipe

Preheat the broiler at 300°F (that is 150°Celsius)
Cut your grapefruit in half and cut it in the form of a
semicircle
Drizzle the top of each grapefruit with honey and 1/8
teaspoon of cinnamon
Broil it for 6 minutes until it starts to brown and serve it
hot.

Nutrients per portion

6 calories
1 g protein
17 carbohydrates

0 g fat
0 mg cholesterol
1 mg sodium
175 mg potassium
1 mg phosphorus
20 mg calcium
1.2 fiber

Hash Brown Omelet

Ingredients

2 tablespoons of diced onion
1 teaspoon of canola oil
2 tablespoons of shredded hash brown
2 tablespoons of diced fresh green bell pepper
1 egg
2 tablespoons soy milk
2 egg whites
2 pieces of parsley

How to prepare the recipe

Heat oil at medium heat and add the diced onion
pieces and green pepper, cooking it for 2 minutes.
Add hash brown and cook it or heat it (if not frozen) for
5 minutes.
Meanwhile, beat the eggs with soy milk and add
nondairy creamer.
Pour the eggs in a pan and cook them to prepare an

omelet until it is ready and firm. Place the hash brown on the omelet in the middle and roll it on a plate. Add parsley and spices.

Nutrients per portion

225 calories
15 g protein
12 g carbohydrates
13 g fat
165 mg cholesterol
180 mg sodium
305 mg potassium
128 mg phosphorus
38 mg calcium
0.9 fiber

Omelet With Apple And Onion

Ingredients

3 eggs
1 water tablespoon
1 butter tablespoon
1 apple
¼ cup of low-fat milk
1/8 tablespoon of black pepper
2 small spoons of cheddar cheese
¾ cup sweet onion

How to prepare the recipe

Peel the apple and slice thinly both apple and onion
Pre heat the over at 400° F (that is around 200°C)
Prepare a small bowl and put in it both water, eggs
with milk, pepper, and leave it there. Melt the butter
over medium heat. Add apple and onion and wait until
the onion becomes translucent for about 5 - 6 minutes.
Spread the mix of onion and apple in the bowl and put
the egg mixture over medium heat until the edges set.
Then add cheddar over the top and put the skillet in
the oven for about 10 minutes.
Divide the omelet into two parts and put it on a plate,
serving it immediately.

Nutrients per portion

284 calories
13 g protein
20 carbohydrates
15 g fat
300 mg cholesterol
165 mg sodium
340 mg potassium
23 mg phosphorus
145 mg calcium
3.5 fiber

Roll Up Burrito

Ingredients

4 eggs
3 tablespoons of green chiles
½ teaspoon of pepper sauce
¼ teaspoon ground cumin
2 flour tortillas in burrito size
Non-stick cooking spray

How to prepare the recipe

Put the non-stick cooking spray in a pan and heat a medium heat.
Beat eggs with green chiles, cumin and hot pepper sauce. Put the eggs into the pan and cook them for 2 minutes.
Heat tortillas in a skillet at medium heat. Place half the eggs mix on each tortilla and roll up.

Nutrients per portion

366 calories
18 g protein
30 g carbohydrates
18 g fat
370 mg cholesterol
590 mg sodium
245 mg potassium
300 mg phosphorus
115 mg calcium
2.5 fiber

Vanilla Waffles

Ingredients

2 eggs
2 glasses of cake flour
¾ glass of low-fat milk
¾ teaspoons of baking soda
¾ cup of sour cream
6 tablespoons of powdered sugar
4 tablespoons of unsalted butter
2 teaspoons of vanilla extract
2 tablespoons of granulated sugar

How to prepare the recipe

Heat the waffle iron
Put together the cake flour and baking soda.
Separate egg whites and yolks. Mix together egg yolks, sour cream, milk and vanilla.
Melt the butter and put it into the sour cream mix.
In another cup beat the egg whites with a hand mixer on medium speed until the peak is soft and add granulated sugar to the egg whites, still beating until stiff peaks form for 3 or 4 minutes.
Beat the sour cream mixture into the flour mix until they combine and then add the egg whites to smooth everything .
Add the batter to the waffle iron, close and cook for

about 3-4 minutes. Serve waffles with powder sugar on it or top it with fresh berries, jam, syrup or whipped cream.

Nutrients per portion

367 calories
8 g protein
50 carbohydrates
15 g fat
98 mg cholesterol
200 mg sodium
150 mg potassium
120 mg phosphorus
80 mg calcium
1 g fiber

Yogurt Fantasy

Ingredients

Greek yogurt
1 spoon of vanilla whey protein powder
½ cup blueberries

How to prepare the recipe

Add protein powder to the yogurt slowly and mix after each addition. Do not mix all at once or it may be clumpy. Wash the blueberries and dry them. Place on top of the yogurt mixture.

Nutrients per portion

185 calories
25 g protein
19 carbohydrates
2 g fat
45 mg cholesterol
122 mg sodium
334 mg potassium
215 mg phosphorus
183 mg calcium
1.8 fiber

Lunch

Fresh Cucumber Soup

Ingredients

2 cucumbers
1/3 cup white onion
1 green onion

1/4 cup fresh mint
2 tablespoons fresh lemon juice
2 tablespoons fresh dill
2/3 cup water
1/3 cup sour cream
1/2 cup half and half cream
1/2 teaspoon pepper
1/4 teaspoon salt

How to prepare the recipe

Remove both peel and seeds from cucumbers.
Cut mint and the onions. Cut up dill.
Put all ingredients in a mixer and whisk until smooth
Cover and place in the refrigerator for at least 2 hour
Use fresh dill sprigs to garnish the soup

Nutrients per portion

78 calories
2 g protein
5 g carbohydrates
5 g fat
11 mg cholesterol
127 mg sodium
257 mg potassium
65 mg phosphorus

Berry Salad With Italian Ricotta Cheese

Ingredients

1 cup of fresh blackberries
1 cup of fresh blueberries
2 cups of fresh strawberry
1/3 cup lemon juice
2 cups of fresh Italian ricotta cheese
1/8 teaspoon of cinnamon

How to prepare the recipe

Wash well both blackberries and blueberries and strawberries. Slice them and put them all together. Add some lemon juice from the cup.
Put the ricotta cheese on a round plate or a bowl and then cover it with berries. Spread the cinnamon on it.

Nutrients per portion

140 calories
15 g protein
15 g carbohydrates
2 g fat
15 mg cholesterol
380 mg sodium
350 mg potassium
180 mg phosphorus
125 mg calcium
4.3 fiber

Celery Tuna Salad

Ingredients
1 piece of celery
15 ounces packed and unsalted tuna
½ apple
½ small onion
2 tablespoons mayonnaise
a bit of black pepper
a little bit of salt

How to prepare the recipe

Prepare the tuna and cut the apple, celery and onion.
Mix all together adding mayonnaise, black pepper and
if you wish some salt.
Serve on lettuce and with unsalted crackers

Nutrients per portion

20 calories
27 g protein
3 g carbohydrates
9 g fat
35 mg cholesterol
185 mg sodium
318 mg potassium

183 mg phosphorus
20 mg calcium
0.8 fiber

Meat Casserole

Ingredients

10 ounces of reduced-fat pork sausage
8 ounces of cream cheese
1 glass of low-fat milk
4 slices of white bread
5 eggs
½ teaspoon dry mustard
½ dry onion flakes

How to prepare the recipe

Preheat oven at 325°F (160°C). Cut the sausage and cook in a cooking dish. Set aside and mix all other ingredients. Add cooked sausage to mixture and place bread pieces in a square casserole, pour sausage mix over the bread and cook for 50 minutes. Cut into 10 portions and serve

Nutrients per portion

222 calories
10 g protein
9 g carbohydrates
15 g fat

145 mg cholesterol
355 mg sodium
200 mg potassium
156 mg phosphorus
96 mg calcium
0.4 fiber

Red And Green Grapes Chicken Salad With Curry

Ingredients
1 apple
1/4 bowl seedless red grapes
1/4 bowl seedless green grapes
4 cooked skinless and boneless chicken breasts
1 piece of celery
1/2 bowl of onion
1/2 bowl of canned water chestnuts
1/2 teaspoon curry powder
3/4 cup mayonnaise
1/8 teaspoon black pepper

How to prepare the recipe

Cut the chicken into small dices and chop celery, onion and apple. Drain and cut chestnuts.
Put together the chicken pieces, celery, onion, apple, grapes, water chestnuts, pepper, curry powder and mayonnaise. Serve it in a big salad bowl.

Nutrients per portion

235 calories
13 g protein
6 g carbohydrates
18 g fat
44 mg cholesterol
160 mg sodium
200 mg potassium
115 mg phosphorus
15 mg calcium
1.1 fiber

Grilled Chicken Pizza

Ingredients

2 pita bread
3 tablespoons low sodium bbq sauce
¼ bowl red onion
4 ounces cooked chicken
2 tablespoons crumbled feta cheese
1/8 teaspoon garlic powder

How to prepare the recipe

Pre heat oven at 350°F (that is 175° C). Place 2 pitas on the pan after you have put non-stick cooking spray on it. Spread bbq sauce (2 tablespoons) on the pita. Cut the onion and put it on pita. Cube chicken and put it on the pitas. Put also both feta and the garlic powder over the pita. Bake for 12 minutes.

Nutrients per portion

320 calories
22 g protein
35 g carbohydrates
9 g fat
50 mg cholesterol
520 mg sodium
250 mg potassium
220 mg phosphorus
160 mg calcium
2.0 fiber

Ground Beef Loan In A Cup

Ingredients

¼ pound ground beef
2 tablespoons of low-fat milk
2 teaspoons of ketchup
2 tablespoons of quick-cooking oats
1 teaspoon onion powder

How to prepare the recipe

Spray a large cup with non-stick cooking spray.
In another cup put together the milk (or its substitute),

ketchup, onion, oats.ù
Crumble meat over the mixture and mix everything, pressing the ground beef.
Cover and put it in the microwave for 3 minutes (high) and serve it very warm.

Nutrients per portion

250 calories
25 g protein
13 g carbohydrates
10 g fat
75 mg cholesterol
160 mg sodium
395 mg potassium
245 mg phosphorus
65 mg calcium
1.4 fiber

Mexican Beef Flour Wrap

Ingredients

5 ounces of cooked roast beef
8 cucumber slices
2 flour Tortillas 6" size
2 tablespoons of whipped cream cheese
2 leaves of light green lettuce
¼ of a bowl of cut red onion

¼ of stripped cut sweet bell pepper
1 teaspoon of herb seasoning blend

How to prepare the recipe

Spread the cheese over the flour wraps. Try to use the ingredients to make two wraps.
Layer the tortillas with roast beef, onions, lettuce, pepper strips and cucumber.
Sprinkle with the herb seasoning. Roll up the wraps and cut them into 4 pieces each. Serve fresh.

Nutrients per portion

255 calories
24 g protein
18 g carbohydrates
10 g fat
70 mg cholesterol
275 mg sodium
445 mg potassium
250 mg phosphorus
58 mg calcium
1.6 fiber

Mixed Chorizo In Egg Flour Wraps

Ingredients

1 pack of chorizo
1 egg
1 flour tortilla or 6" size

How to prepare the recipe

Cook the chorizo in a pan on stove, cutting the meat into small pieces.
Eliminate excessive water or fat and add 1 egg combining all while they are being cooked.
Serve everything on a flour tortilla or wrapping the tortillas.

Nutrients per portion

223 calories
15 g protein
15 g carbohydrates
11 g fat
210 mg cholesterol
315 mg sodium
285 mg potassium
230 mg phosphorus
78 mg calcium
1.5 fiber

Sandwich With Chicken Salad

Ingredients

2 bowls of cooked chicken
½ cup of low-fat mayonnaise
½ cup of green bell pepper
1 cup of pieces of pineapple
1/3 cup of carrots
4 slices of flatbread
½ teaspoon of black pepper

How to prepare the recipe

Prepare aside the diced chicken and drain pineapple, adding green bell pepper , black pepper and carrots. Combine all in a bowl and refrigerate until chilled. Later on, serve the chicken salad on the flatbread.

Nutrients per portion

345 calories
22 g protein
24 g carbohydrates
15 g fat
60 mg cholesterol
395 mg sodium
330 mg potassium
165 mg phosphorus

15 mg calcium
1.5 fiber

Spice Bread With Tuna Salad

Ingredients

1 tablespoon of onion
1 piece of celery
1 fresh tomato
Some lettuce leaves
1 tablespoon low calories mayonnaise
1 medium bagel or spiced bread
½ pack low sodium of water-packed canned tuna

How to prepare the recipe

Chop onion, tomato and celery. Open tuna and cut it into small pieces. Put everything in the bagel on the lettuce leaves adding some mayonnaise and close the spiced bread.

Nutrients per portion

290 calories
25 g protein
30 g carbohydrates
7 g fat
20 mg cholesterol

475 mg sodium
320 mg potassium
175 mg phosphorus
15 mg calcium
2.5 g fiber

Smoothie With Lemon

Ingredients

4 teaspoons of sugar substitute
2 teaspoons of lemon juice
3 tablespoons whipped topping
8 ounces pasteurized liquid egg white

How to prepare the recipe

Put together all ingredients. Mix until the topping melts together well.

Nutrients per portion

225 calories
28 g protein
22 g carbohydrates
3 g fat
0 mg cholesterol
425 mg sodium
430 mg potassium
35 mg phosphorus

19 mg calcium
0 g fiber

Stuffed Omelet

Ingredients

2 tablespoons of red bell chopped pepper
2 tablespoons of orange bell chopped pepper
2 tablespoons of chopped green onion
2 tablespoons of fresh sliced mushrooms
1 teaspoon of chopped garlic
1 tablespoon butter
1 tablespoon canola oil
2 eggs
2 egg whites
4 tablespoon 1% low-fat milk
1/8 teaspoon ground cumin
1/8 teaspoon pepper

How to prepare the recipe

Pass the vegetables with garlic in butter or in oil mixture until they are tenderly crispy. Mix up eggs, egg whites and milk until they are light and tender as well. Mix it in cumin and pepper and pour egg mixture over the vegetables.
Reduce heat and cover for 1 to 2 minutes. Uncover and after egg is completely cooked, fold omelet over in the

pan. Divide the omelet into 2 portions and serve. You can also garnish with green onion or a mushroom slice.

Nutrients per portion

220 calories
12 g protein
4 g carbohydrates
1 g fat
203 mg cholesterol
185 mg sodium
245 mg potassium
145 mg phosphorus
81 mg calcium
1.0 fiber

Tiny Rice Pies

Ingredients

Vegetable oil (2 tablespoons)
1 teaspoon of mustard seeds
Half cup of semolina
2 green finely cut chilies
1/8 teaspoon salt
¼ cup of yogurt
¼ glass of water
¼ grated corn
¼ Indian cheese

Some bits of finely cut cilandro
1 tablespoon of clarified butter

How to prepare the recipe

Heat the oil and the seeds in a pan and add semolina, chilies and a bit of salt. Cook it until the semolina becomes a bit brown. Let it cool down. Put together yogurt with some water and mix it until it is smooth, then add corn, Indian cheese, cilantro, yogurt and add everything to semolina, leaving it aside for 10-15 minutes.
Put the clarified butter in a pan, steaming then the semolina mix for 10 minutes.
Put some cilantro on the semolina circles and serve them still a bit warm.

Nutrients per portion

175 calories
5 g protein
14 g carbohydrates
10 g fat
4 mg cholesterol
214 mg sodium
140 mg potassium
89 mg phosphorus

65 mg calcium
0.8 fiber

Toast Topped With Creamy Eggs

Ingredients

4 slices white bread
6 eggs
4 ounces cream cheese
3 tablespoons of unsalted butter
1/3 cup flour
1-1/2 cups unsweetened, plain almond milk
1/2 tablespoon of yellow mustard
1/8 teaspoon pepper

How to prepare the recipe

Hard boil the eggs for 12 minutes. Remove them from heat, drain and cover with cool water. Peel and chop boiled eggs. Put together the butter and flour in a sauce pan at medium low heat. Mix constantly until well combined.
Add almond milk, cream cheese, mustard and pepper to butter and flour mixture. Let it thicken and add the eggs to the sauce, keeping at a warm heat. Toast the bread and put the egg mixture over the toast before serving.

Nutrients per portion

430 calories
15 g protein
25 g carbohydrates
28 g fat
330 mg cholesterol
400 mg sodium
250 mg potassium
210 mg phosphorus
220 mg calcium
1.6 fiber

Dinner

Chicken With Vegetables And Worcestershire Sauce

Ingredients

1 cup of frozen sliced carrots
1 cup of frozen green beans
½ cup of diced onion
1 pound chicken breasts (boneless and skinless)
½ cup low sodium chicken consommé
Worcestershire sauce (2 teaspoons)
1 small spoon of herb seasoning

How to prepare the recipe

Put together carrots, green beans and onion in a pan and cook them slowly. Put the chicken breasts on vegetables and pour the consommé over the chicken. Top with Worcestershire sauce and herb seasoning. Cook at a high heat for 3 hours or low heat for 6 hours. Serve the chicken accompanied by the consommé in a cup and the vegetable mix.

Nutrients per portion

180 calories
25 g protein
10 g carbohydrates
3 g fat
70 mg cholesterol
185 mg sodium
430 mg potassium
225 mg phosphorus
55 mg calcium
3.2 fiber

Ground Beef Soup

Ingredients

Lean ground beef cut in small balls (1 pound)
½ glass of onion
1 small spoon seasoning and browning sauce
2 small spoons of lemon pepper seasoning blend
Some reduced-sodium beef consommé

2 glasses of water
Half dish white rice
Half pack of frozen mixed vegetables (corn, carrots, peas, beans and green beans)
Half spoon of sour cream

How to prepare the recipe

Brown ground beef with cut onion in a pan and eliminate fat. Add seasoning sauce, water, consommé, rice and vegetables. On high heat boil the ingredients and after lowering the heat, cook for 30 minutes.
Put the meatballs in the consommé and cook at a low heat still for half an hour until ready to serve.

Nutrients per portion

220 calories
20 g protein
18 g carbohydrates
8 g fat
50 mg cholesterol
170 mg sodium
445 mg potassium
210 mg phosphorus
42 mg calcium
4.2 fiber

Ground Turkey Burger

Ingredients

1 pound ground lean turkey
6 hamburger buns
½ dish red onion
½ dish of green bell pepper
1 half spoon of chicken grilled blend seasoning
2 small spoons of brown sugar
1 tablespoon Worcestershire sauce
1 cup of low sodium tomato sauce

How to prepare the recipe

Cook the turkey at medium heat. Cut little pieces of onion and green bell pepper. Mix the sauce, the grilled blend seasoning and tomato sauce. Add seasoning to the turkey mixture and cook for 10 minutes. Prepare 5 portions and put in burger buns.

Nutrients per portion

28 calories
24 g protein
28 g carbohydrates
9 g fat
55 mg cholesterol
285 mg sodium
510 mg potassium
235 mg phosphorus
85 mg calcium
1.8 fiber

One Portion Frittatas

Ingredients

4 eggs
2 tablespoons red bell pepper
2 tablespoons green bell pepper
2 tablespoons onion
2 ounces cooked lean ham
1 tablespoon low-fat milk
1 pound frozen hash brown potatoes
½ bowl low-fat cheddar cheese
Black pepper

* How to prepare the recipe

Put the potatoes in water in a bowl for 4 hours.
Eliminate excessive water.
Pre heat oven at 375°F (or 200°C). Coat 8 muffin tins
holes with cooking spray. Put hash brown potatoes in
the tins and press them in the bottom then spray also
the potatoes with cooking spray. Cook for 12-15
minutes at 350°F (175° C). Cut the ham, pepper and
onion finely and beat both milk and eggs together in a
bowl. Season with pepper and add ham, pepper, onion
and cheese to the mixture.
Put the hash brown potatoes in the muffin holes
pressing them and out ¼ bowl egg mixture in the

center of each muffin hole. Put again the pan in the oven and let the potatoes become crispy in about 15 to 20 minutes.

Once ready, let the muffins sit on a dish for 5 minutes before serving.

Nutrients per portion

110 calories
8 g protein
10 g carbohydrates
4 g fat
100 mg cholesterol
115 mg sodium
160 mg potassium
130 mg phosphorus
52 mg calcium
1.0 fiber

Pan Fried Beef And Broccoli

Ingredients

2 garlic small slices
1 tomato
8 ounces uncooked lean sirloin beef
12 ounces of frozen broccoli stir fry vegetable blend

2 little spoons of peanut oil
¼ cup low sodium chicken consommé
1 small spoon of cornstarch
2 little spoons of reduced-sodium soy sauce
2 bowls of cooked rice

How to prepare the recipe

Cut the garlic cloves and tomato. Cut the beef into strips and place the broccoli in the microwave for 3-4 minutes. In a wok pan heat oil and the garlic to make them fragrant. Add vegetable blend cooking it for about 4 minutes or more and remove from pan.
Add the beef in the same pot and cook it for around 7-8 minutes, then prepare the sauce putting together the consommé, the soy sauce and cornstarch.
Add vegetables, sauce, tomato and heat them with the beef until the sauce is ready. Serve the dish with brown rice.

Nutrients per portion

370 calories
18 g protein
35 g carbohydrates
17 g fat
40 mg cholesterol
350 mg sodium
550 mg potassium
250 mg phosphorus

60 mg calcium
5.1 fiber

Pork Chops And Apples

Ingredients

Unsalted margarine (2 tablespoons)
6 ounces of low sodium stuffing mix for chicken
20 ounces apple pie filling
6 boneless pork loin chops
Olive oil

How to prepare the recipe

Put a baking pan in the oven at 350°F (or 200°C) and grease it with olive oil.
Put together the stuffing and mix it in water and margarine. Spread the apple pie pieces on the bottom of the pan and place pork chops on it. Put the stuffing on top of pork chops.
Cover with parchment paper and bake for 30 minutes. Remove the paper and still leave it in the oven for 10 minutes.

Nutrients per portion

490 calories
25 g protein
45 g carbohydrates
20 g fat
55 mg cholesterol

365 mg sodium
405 mg potassium
220 mg phosphorus
25 mg calcium
1.0 fiber

www.ingramcontent.com/pod-product-compliance
Lightning Source LLC
Chambersburg PA
CBHW062137020426
42335CB00013B/1243